Fast Facts

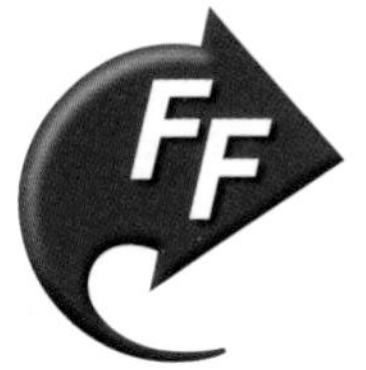

Fast Facts: Dementia

Second edition

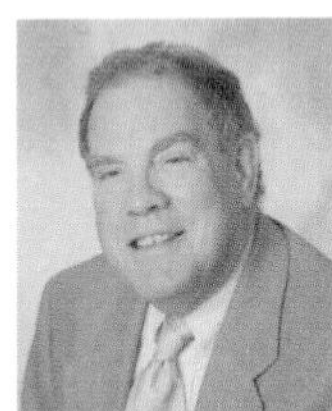

Lawrence J Whalley MD FRCPsych FRCP(E)
Professor of Mental Health
University of Aberdeen Clinical Research Centre
Royal Cornhill Hospital
Aberdeen, UK

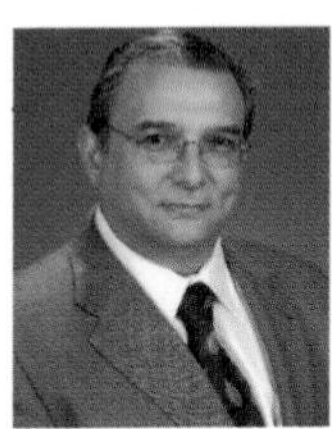

John CS Breitner MD MPH
Director, Genetic Research Education and Clinical Center
VA Puget Sound Health Care System
Professor, Department of Psychiatry and
Behavioral Sciences
University of Washington School of Medicine
Seattle, Washington, USA

Declaration of Independence
This book is as balanced and as practical as we can make it.
Ideas for improvement are always welcome: feedback@fastfacts.com

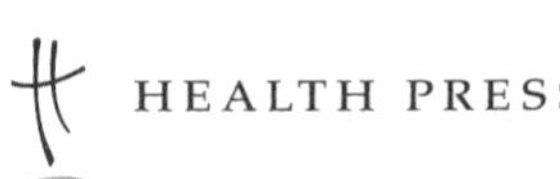
HEALTH PRESS

Fast Facts: Dementia
First published 2002
Second edition November 2009

Health Press Limited, Elizabeth House, Queen Street, Abingdon,
Oxford OX14 3LN, UK
Tel: +44 (0)1235 523233
Fax: +44 (0)1235 523238

Book orders can be placed by telephone or via the website.
For regional distributors or to order via the website, please go to:
www.fastfacts.com
For telephone orders, please call +44 (0)1752 202301 (UK and Europe),
1 800 247 6553 (USA, toll free), +1 419 281 1802 (Americas)
or +61 (0)2 9698 7755 (Asia–Pacific).

A CIP record for this title is available from the British Library.

ISBN 978-1-903734-17-9

Whalley LJ (Lawrence)
Fast Facts: Dementia/
Lawrence J Whalley, John CS Breitner

Medical illustrations by Dee McLean, London, UK.
Typesetting and page layout by Zed, Oxford, UK.
Printed by Latimer Trend & Company Limited, Plymouth, UK.

Text printed with vegetable inks on biodegradable and recyclable paper manufactured using elemental chlorine free (ECF) wood pulp from well-managed forests.

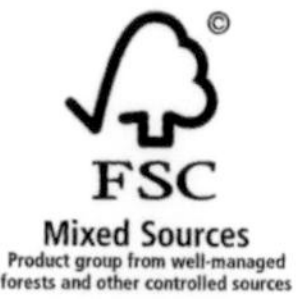

Glossary of abbreviations

ACh: acetylcholine

AChE: acetylcholinesterase

ACTH: adrenocorticotropic hormone

ADL: activities of daily living

APP: amyloid precursor protein

ChAT: choline acetyltransferase

DSM-IV: *Diagnostic and Statistical Manual of Mental Disorders*, fourth edition

DSRS: Dementia Symptom Rating Scale

DZ: dizygotic [twin]

GABA: gamma-aminobutyric acid

ICD-10: *International Statistical Classification of Diseases and Related Health Problems*, tenth revision

MAP: microtubule-associated protein

MMSE: mini mental state examination

MRI: magnetic resonance imaging

MZ: monozygotic [twin]

NART: National Adult Reading Test

NFT: neurofibrillary tangle

NMDA: *N*-methyl-D-aspartate

NPI: Neuropsychiatric Inventory

NSAID: non-steroidal anti-inflammatory drug

PET: positron emission tomography

PHF: paired helical filament

ROS: reactive oxygen species

SPECT: single photon emission computerized tomography

Introduction

Whenever one of us lectures publically about dementia, someone in the audience is almost certain to ask, 'Is dementia the same as Alzheimer's disease?' And almost as often, someone will ask, 'What's the difference between ordinary forgetfulness in old age and dementia?' Or, 'Doesn't everyone get dementia if they live long enough?' Our answers are straightforward: Alzheimer's disease is one of the causes of dementia but there are many other less common causes. Dementia is different from normal age-related forgetfulness, both because memory loss is more severe and because other abilities such as language are affected. We don't really know the answer to the last question, so our carefully worded reply usually prompts more questions about the true nature of the dementias of old age. If pressed, we point to the typical degenerative changes that characteristically accompany most dementing illnesses, and we note that these changes almost always affect key brain areas that are critical for memory ('bottle-neck structures').

Nowadays, after enormous research efforts, it is true to say that more is known about the cause, course and treatment of the dementias than about any other psychiatric disorder. However, one research goal that remains unfulfilled – and is still a major worry and priority for many old people, public health doctors and politicians – is the early recognition of dementia, or more accurately the recognition of early dementia. Many predict that if dementia is ever to be prevented we will need the ability to identify patients at the very early stages of their illness or – better yet – those who are at greatest risk but who lack overt symptoms. So far, no hard and fast rules can reliably define the dementia 'prodrome'. Instead, the idea gaining currency is that the brain possesses 'cognitive reserve' ('brain reserve' or 'neural reserve') that enables it to withstand or buffer the presence of the early brain changes of dementia. Close study suggests that, like dementia itself, reserve consists of diverse parts that include education, original mental ability, accumulated stressful experiences and much more. If such reserve can be shown to have a sound biological basis, this discovery may lead to interventions and suggest novel approaches to the delay of dementia.

The holistic care of a person with dementia encompasses health and social elements. In developed societies, both have improved markedly over the past decades. In the USA, and possibly elsewhere in the developed world, there are established trends towards lower rates of disability and decreased mortality (especially among men) from acute myocardial infarction. These improvements attest to the impact of many innovations in risk factor reduction in primary and geriatric specialty care. These developments have relevance to dementia care.

First, public health strategies that lessen exposure to vascular risk factors reduce the frequency of acute vascular events. Examples include better control of hypertension, diabetes and lifestyle factors. In this sense, the association between mid-life vascular risk factors and late-onset dementia emerges as the single greatest opportunity to reduce the occurrence of dementia among the elderly.

Second, progress in social care of the elderly provides a sound basis for the claim that dementia care is improving, that quality of life is getting better and that, in step with improved geriatric care, the outlook for the elderly, including those with cognitive disabilities and dementia has improved. In time, these steps forward will lengthen with the growth of scientific knowledge. At present we are passing through a mature phase in the development of dementia services. We know that at our best what we do for persons with dementia can show our capacity for compassion to advantage, and that our standards of care help safeguard not only our own liberal values but also the independence of those with dementia.

This fully updated second edition of *Fast Facts: Dementia* begins with a review of the basic neuroscience, followed by a discussion of brain aging and its relationship to neurodegenerative disease. It then considers the cause, course and treatment of the common illnesses that can provoke dementia syndrome. Our aim is to equip the primary care physician and other members of the healthcare team with an understanding of the basic causes of dementia, particularly Alzheimer's disease, the clinical characteristics of dementia, and the basic principles of its evaluation and management. We hope that, in the process, readers will learn some of the steps that will improve the long-term care of patients with dementia or perhaps even prevent dementia.

1 Basic neuroscience

Although the presence of dementia does not always imply the existence of an identifiable brain disease, it usually does so. A basic knowledge of some of the principles of neuroscience and the anatomy and physiology of the brain is therefore essential to a basic understanding of dementing illness.

Simple functional anatomy of the brain

An adult human brain weighs approximately 1.3 kg. The central nervous system of the adult brain is divided into six main parts: the spinal cord; the medulla, pons and midbrain that together comprise the brainstem; the diencephalon; and the two cerebral hemispheres (Figure 1.1).

The largest components are the two cerebral hemispheres, which are principally responsible for the higher intellectual functions that distinguish humans from non-human primates. They consist of the cerebral cortex and three deep-lying structures:

- the basal ganglia, involved with regulation of activity and motor performance
- the hippocampi (singular hippocampus), involved with memory
- the amygdaloid nuclei, involved with linkage of nervous and hormonal responses to emotions.

Deeper and older in evolutionary terms are the diencephalon and brainstem. The diencephalon contains two structures:

- the thalamus, which acts principally as a relay station for information passing to the cerebral cortex from the rest of the nervous system
- the hypothalamus, which regulates hormonal, autonomic and other basic body functions such as temperature control, salt and water balance, thirst and appetite.

Within the brainstem, the midbrain controls many sensory and motor functions such as eye movements and coordination of visual and auditory reflexes. Nerve tracts in the pons convey information about movement from the cerebral hemispheres to the cerebellum, which

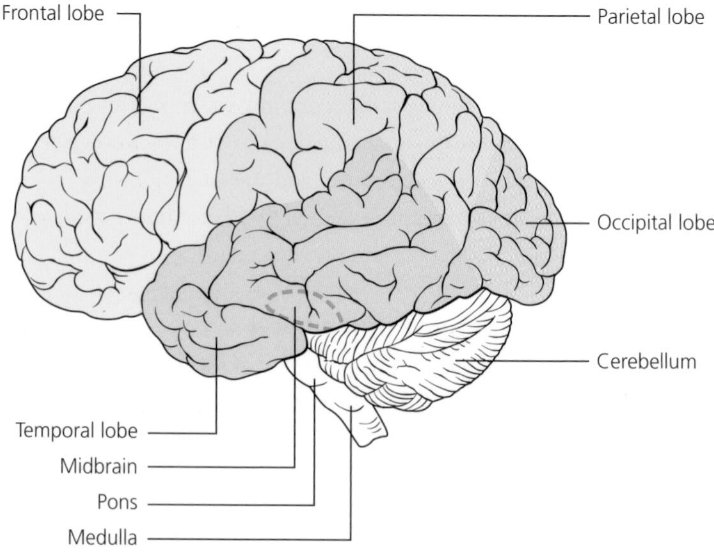

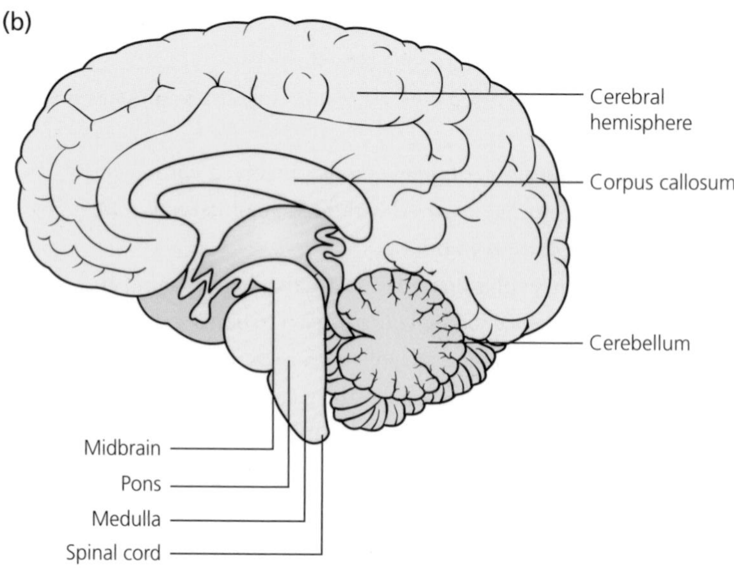

Figure 1.1 Schematic views of the brain: (a) lateral view; (b) midsagittal section.

modulates and integrates the force and range of muscle movements. Nerve centers in the medulla control digestion, breathing and heart rate.

Early studies of patients with strokes or other focal brain injuries revealed that different brain regions contribute to distinct mental abilities and functions. For example, the frontal lobes are mainly concerned with planning future actions, controlling movements and the abilities associated with self-monitoring and abstract reasoning. The parietal lobes are instrumental in somatic sensation and body image, and in visuospatial reasoning. The occipital lobes are devoted largely to vision. The temporal lobes, which are especially often affected by dementing illness, are important for learning and memory, language functions and emotional responses. However, 'parallel processing' is an important organizational principle of brain function. The term implies that when a region or pathway is damaged others may be able to compensate partly for the loss.

Brain cells

In the 19th and early 20th centuries, pioneering neuroanatomists and neuropathologists studied the structures of the brain using careful light microscopy techniques. They identified two characteristic cell types in the brain: neurons (Figure 1.2) and neuroglia.

Neurons, like all cells, are contained within a lipid-bilayer membrane. The fatty acid components of the membrane are oriented with their lipid 'tails' facing inwards towards the opposite layer. Large protein molecules span or are embedded in the membrane and allow structural communication between neurons, and may also be receptors for neurotransmitters or other chemicals that affect cell function. Without such specific 'gateways', drugs must be lipid-soluble to enter brain cells, and hence their rate of entry into the brain depends on their lipid solubility.

Neurons usually have one long process, the axon, which connects with neurons at some distance. They also have many other processes called dendrites that extend like the branches of a tree away from the cell body of the neuron. These dendritic branches receive connections

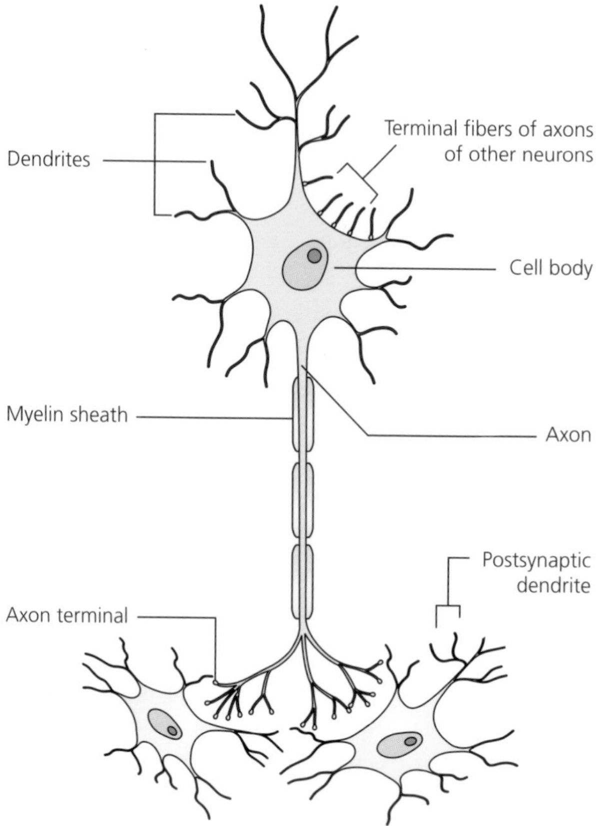

Figure 1.2 Structure of a typical neuron, showing points of contact with cell bodies, axons and dendrites of other neurons.

from other nearby neurons, or from other more distant neurons via lengthy axons.

Internal cell structure. In addition to components common to all cells, neurons have within their cytoplasm several types of membrane pockets, called vesicles or vacuoles depending on their shape and size. Vesicles often contain chemical neurotransmitters and are typically concentrated close to a synapse ready to release their contents (Figure 1.3). Also, protein threads within the cytoplasm, called microfilaments, function primarily as a supportive system.

Microtubules, distinct from microfilaments, are hollow cylindrical protein structures within the cell cytoplasm that:

- provide the cytoskeleton
- help neurons extend long axonal and dendritic processes
- have an important role in transport of materials within the cell, particularly to distant points at the ends of axons and dendrites.

The proteins involved in the assembly of microtubules, called microtubule-associated proteins (MAPs), are abnormal in Alzheimer's disease. Some mutations of the *MAPT* (also known as *TAU*) gene can provoke neurodegenerative dementias.

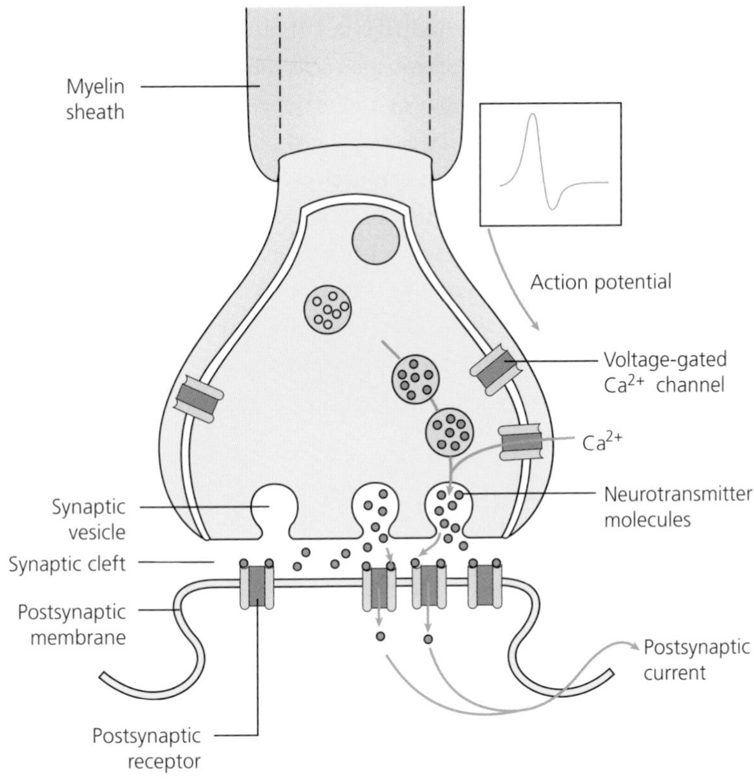

Figure 1.3 Basic mechanism of neurotransmission at a typical synapse.

Cell-surface molecules. Large regulatory biomolecules studded in neuron cell membranes are crucial for transfer of information between brain cells and in cell–cell adhesion and recognition. They include:

- amyloid precursor protein (APP), a large protein that spans the cell surface membrane and appears to be important in the biology of Alzheimer's disease
- receptors, large cell-surface molecules that recognize chemical transmitters released from adjacent neurons. Each receptor recognizes only one type of neurotransmitter but there may be more than one type of receptor for a single neurotransmitter.

Neuroglia. There are three principal types of glia in the brain.

Astroglia (astrocytes) are star-shaped cells thought to have a supporting role in the development and maintenance of the nervous system. They also appear to have crucial tasks in the provision of molecular signals to organize brain cell growth, differentiation and repair, and in the organization of brain response to injury.

Microglia are small round scavenger cells that prepare unwanted material for immune elimination and then remove it, much as macrophages function outside the blood–brain barrier.

Schwann cells are specialized for the production of myelin, the fatty insulation that surrounds the long axons of some larger neurons.

Synapses

Communication between adjacent neurons occurs at cell–cell junctions called synapses (see Figure 1.3). Brain cells make complex patterns of synaptic connections to form local neural networks, which link together to perform essential brain tasks such as memory or language. These networks adapt to experience by changing the structure and efficiency of their connections. This adaptation process, known as 'synaptic plasticity', is described at the end of this chapter (see page 17).

Early neuroscientists recognized the importance of synapses and thought that they acted like wiring contacts, passing information in the form of electrical pulses between nerve cells. We now know that electrical synaptic transmission occurs rarely in the nervous system and that most synapses pass information using chemical signals called neurotransmitters. These fall into two large groups: 'classic' neurotransmitters and peptide neurotransmitters, described below.

'Classic' neurotransmitters

The so-called classic, or small-molecule, neurotransmitters are contained within vesicles that are typically concentrated close to a synapse, ready to release their contents into the synaptic cleft (see Figure 1.3). These neurotransmitters can have varied effects, either exciting or inhibiting the activity of the target postsynaptic cell. Neurons are often classified by the type of neurotransmitter they use to send their signals: for example, cells that transmit signals using the neurotransmitter dopamine are called dopaminergic neurons; those that use histamine are called histaminergic neurons, and so on. The following small-molecule neurotransmitters are among those implicated in the pathophysiology of brain disorders.

Gamma-aminobutyric acid (GABA) functions mainly as an inhibitory neurotransmitter; approximately half of the brain's cells use it. Disturbance in GABA function can produce devastating effects such as epilepsy.

Glutamate is the principal excitatory neurotransmitter in the brain. Cells that receive glutamate signals can be overstimulated and die (excitotoxicity). Excitotoxic cell death is thought to be an important cause of neurodegeneration in several brain diseases, including Huntington's disease, and it may have a role in the dementias of aging such as Alzheimer's disease and vascular dementia.

Dopamine is an excitatory neurotransmitter that sends signals to higher structures from the brainstem. These signals are important regulators of activity level in their target areas. Dysregulation of dopaminergic transmission is also an important cause of 'psychotic' symptoms such as hallucinations or delusions that are characteristic of schizophrenia but are also found in patients with dementia.

Norepinephrine (noradrenaline) and serotonin are small-molecule neurotransmitters that are also synthesized in discrete areas of the brainstem. Axonal projections from these areas extend to large regions of the diencephalon and cortex, where their synaptic activity regulates mood and various behavioral 'drive' phenomena.

Acetylcholine (ACh) has a more specialized function. The cells that synthesize this neurotransmitter have their cell bodies in specific deep brain structures, including the nucleus basalis of Meynert (a part of the medial basal forebrain) and adjacent regions. Their axons project extensively to many higher brain structures such as the cortex and hippocampi, where the level of transmitter release probably has an important influence on other neural systems, such as those critical for memory and cognition (Figure 1.4). Cholinergic activity is characteristically impaired in Alzheimer's disease.

Cholinergic neurotransmission. ACh is stored in vesicles at the terminal of a presynaptic cholinergic neuron. When the cell fires, depolarization of the presynaptic terminal membrane opens voltage-dependent calcium channels. Calcium mediates the fusion of vesicles with the presynaptic membrane, resulting in release of ACh into the synaptic cleft by a process called exocytosis (Figure 1.5). The transmitter molecules then attach to cholinergic receptors on the postsynaptic membrane of an adjacent neuron.

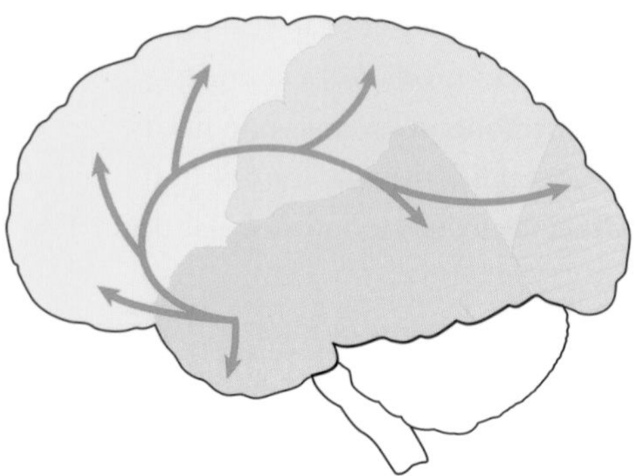

Figure 1.4 Cholinergic projections to the cerebral cortex from the brainstem.

Depending on the nature of the receptor, this binding of transmitter can result in several processes (see below). Free or bound ACh is quickly broken down by the enzyme acetylcholinesterase into choline and acetate (or the free neurotransmitter may diffuse away into a nearby astrocyte). The choline is mostly reabsorbed into the presynaptic terminal, where it is reprocessed into ACh. There are two types of cholinergic receptors: muscarinic receptors and nicotinic receptors.

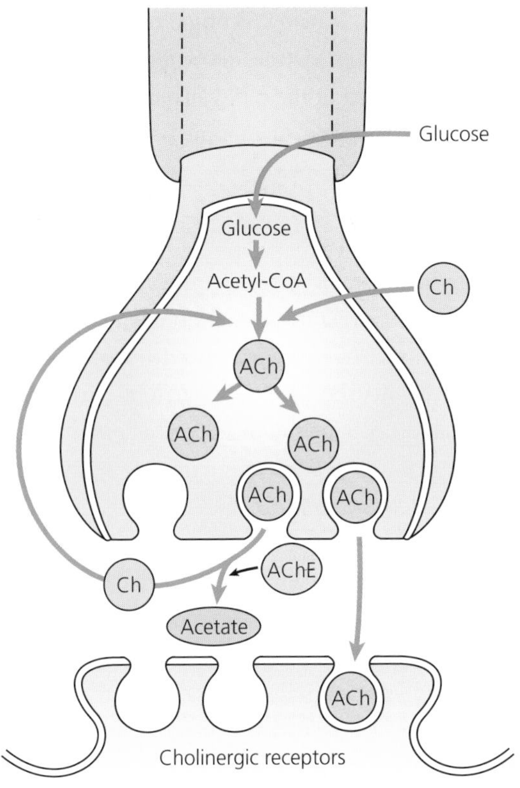

Figure 1.5 Neurotransmission at cholinergic synapses, showing the role of acetylcholinesterase (AChE) in breaking down acetylcholine (ACh) into choline (Ch) and acetate.

Muscarinic receptors bind ACh but differ from other cholinergic receptors in that they also react to the quaternary amine muscarine and can be blocked by atropine. Muscarinic receptors belong to the class of metabotropic receptors, the activation of which results in activation of a 'second messenger' protein within the cell, which in turn releases intracellular calcium and opens nearby potassium channels.

Nicotinic receptors differ from muscarinic cholinergic receptors in that they are activated not only by ACh but also by nicotine, and are not blocked by atropine. When a nicotinic receptor complex is activated, it changes shape and charge, allowing ions to pass directly from the outside to the inside of the cell. Current then spreads to adjacent areas of the postsynaptic membrane – which contributes to depolarization of the membrane.

Peptide neurotransmitters

Rather than responding to small-molecule transmitters, some metabotropic receptors bind peptides, or short chains of amino acids that are the building blocks of larger proteins. Until about 25 years ago it was thought that each neuron used only one type of transmitter. However, Hokfeldt and colleagues in Sweden then established the principle of 'coexistence'. They observed that nerve cells could contain both a small-molecule 'classic' neurotransmitter and a peptide neurotransmitter.

Peptide neurotransmitters usually have specialized functions restricted to particular brain areas. They were first discovered to regulate the release of various hormones by these brain areas, but it is now clear that they also have more widespread importance. They are present typically at concentrations about 1000-fold lower than the 'classic' transmitters, and are intimately involved in the regulation of the latter's release. Their names often derive from their endocrine actions: for example, somatostatin inhibits growth hormone and corticotropin-releasing factor stimulates the release of adrenocorticotropic hormone. Levels of some peptide neurotransmitters are substantially reduced in Alzheimer's disease, and some treatments have been based on attempts to replace them.

Synaptic plasticity

Patterns of connections between brain cells are not rigid and unchanging. Instead, they are in a constant state of rearrangement – a phenomenon called 'synaptic plasticity'. Early in brain development there is overproduction of synapses, which are then reduced in number in early adolescence by a process called 'synaptic pruning'. Much later in life there is a more gradual and insidious loss of synapses. It is unclear whether this loss results from a much slower form of the same sort of 'pruning' mechanism.

The precise implications of the changes in number of synapses with aging are unknown. However, reduction in synaptic density may reduce the capacity of the brain to respond to experience. There is evidence that synaptic plasticity underpins brain processes as different as memory and brain repair after injury. The brain mechanisms that determine normal development of the nervous system are also thought to be involved in the determination and regulation of synaptic plasticity.

To achieve a perfect relationship between brain information processing and rearrangement of synapses, electrical impulses must be able to influence, in a very precise manner, long-term changes in local neuronal circuit architecture and function. This is probably achieved by regulation of the expression of specific DNA sequences inside the neuronal nucleus. In turn, expression of DNA modifies the production of local tropic factors, or the responsiveness of nearby cells to them. These mechanisms probably allow a local group of neurons to 'remember' their exact excitatory or inhibitory patterns of input.

Synaptic plasticity is currently the best hypothesis to explain human memory. Failure to maintain synaptic plasticity as a part of brain aging (or possibly 'pruning' losses of synaptic density) may produce the memory problems typical of healthy (non-pathological) old age, as well as some of the early features of dementia. Although synaptic plasticity is generally thought to be a 'necessary' component of memory, it is not established whether on its own it provides sufficient explanation for memory. Future interventions for the treatment of dementia will probably be designed to retain or strengthen the biological mechanisms of synaptic plasticity.

Key points – basic neuroscience

- There are two types of brain cells: neurons and glia. Neurons do brain work; they process information. Glia support and protect neurons and may modulate their work.
- Neurons communicate at synapses. The functions of many synapses and patterns of connections are modified in a process called synaptic plasticity.
- Most synapses communicate using a chemical transmitter. Acetylcholine is one such transmitter. It supports brain functions that include learning and memory.
- Peptide neurotransmitters have specialized functions restricted to particular brain areas; they may modify the effects of the classic neurotransmitters.
- The surface of a neuron contains many large molecules involved in cell–cell recognition and adhesion. One of these, the amyloid precursor protein, appears to be important in the biology of Alzheimer's disease.
- The internal structure of the neuron is supported by a microtubular cytoskeleton. Special proteins that help assemble the cytoskeleton (microtubule-associated proteins) are abnormal in Alzheimer's disease.

Key references

Arshavsky YI. "The seven sins" of the Hebbian synapse: can the hypothesis of synaptic plasticity explain long-term memory consolidation? *Prog Neurobiol* 2006;80:99–113.

Bruel-Jungerman E, Davis S, Laroche S. Brain plasticity mechanisms and memory: a party of four. *Neuroscientist* 2007; 13:492–505.

Dan Y, Poo MM. Spike timing-dependent plasticity: from synapse to perception. *Physiol Rev* 2006; 86:1033–48.

Eriksson PS, Perfilieva E, Bjork-Eriksson T et al. Neurogenesis in the adult hippocampus. *Nat Med* 1998; 4:1313–17.

Goda Y, Davis GW. Mechanisms of synapse assembly and disassembly. *Neuron* 2003;40:243–64.

Kandel ER, Schwartz JH, Jessell TM. *Essentials of Neural Science and Behavior.* Englewood Cliffs, NJ: Prentice Hall, 1995.

Kolb B, Whishaw IQ. *Fundamentals of Human Neuropsychology*, 3rd edn. New York: WH Freeman and Co., 1990.

Maletic-Savatic M, Malinow R, Svoboda K. Rapid dendritic morphogenesis in CA1 hippocampal dendrites induced by synaptic activity. *Science* 1999;283:1923–7.

Mayford M. Protein kinase signaling in synaptic plasticity and memory. *Curr Opin Neurobiol* 2007;17: 313–17.

Speese SD, Budnik V. Wnts: up-and-coming at the synapse. *Trends Neurosci* 2007;30:268–75.

2 The aging brain

Anatomy and chemistry of the aging brain

Because dementia occurs most often in old age, it is important to understand several brain changes that occur with aging, and which of these result from normal physiological brain aging and which from dementing illnesses.

Brain shrinkage. At about 50 years of age, the brain begins to shrink from an average weight of 1.3 kg to about 1.2 kg by 65 years of age. Contrary to widespread belief, this shrinkage does not reflect a generalized loss of nerve cells. It results from loss of water, and reductions in the 'normal' complement of brain cells in a few specific areas of the brain ('selective neuronal loss'). This type of selective loss of brain substance is nearly universal in aging, but atrophy is much more striking in the presence of age-related neurodegenerative disease.

As the brain shrinks with age, the gaps between folds of the cortex (sulci) widen and the spaces (ventricles) inside the brain enlarge. In Alzheimer's disease, this cortical shrinkage is more extensive and may be more marked in specific local regions such as the temporal or parietal areas. It is not known whether the changes of Alzheimer's disease are categorically distinct from those of 'normal' aging, or whether they represent an exaggeration of these changes.

Magnetic resonance imaging (MRI) reveals the distribution of water in brain tissue and can thus be used to detect brain shrinkage. The image thus provides a model of water distribution in the brain, and MRI-based maps of normal brain aging are available. These show the need for great care in the interpretation of MRI scans of aging brains (Figure 2.1). In addition to showing water distribution, MRI scans also reveal brain structures in great detail. They show individual skull bones (as in an X-ray), the gray matter of the cortex and subcortical nuclei, and the white matter tracts that connect areas of cortical gray matter with each other and with other brain structures.

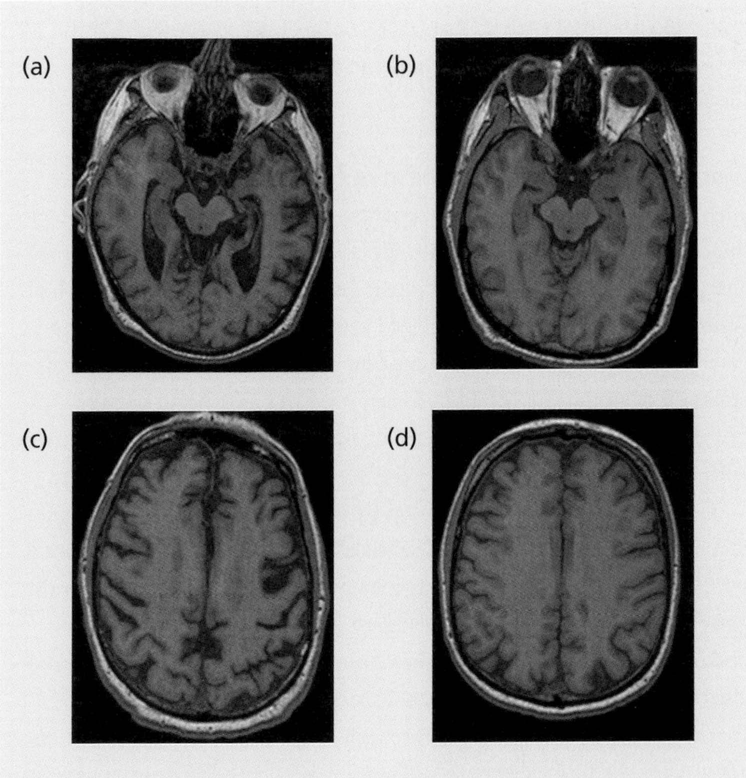

Figure 2.1 MRI scans of normal and pathologically atrophied brains. Scans (a) and (c) show sulcal widening and/or enlarged ventricles compared with the brains of normal controls shown in scans (b) and (d), respectively. Images reproduced courtesy of Dr A Murray, Aberdeen Royal Infirmary, UK.

MRI data can be analyzed using a special technique called diffusion tensor imaging to reveal the fine structure of bundles of white matter fibers (Figure 2.1a).

Synaptic and neuronal loss. Coleman and Flood carefully reviewed studies on brain cell loss with aging and challenged the validity of the consensus view that brain aging in the absence of dementia is related to brain cell death. Later studies showed that, in the absence of dementia, there was no neuronal loss from two brain structures that are particularly affected by Alzheimer's disease: the hippocampus and the entorhinal cortex. Robert Terry has instead shown that the basis of the functional deficits in dementia may be the structural loss of synapses.

Glucose consumption. The work done by the brain also decreases with age. Although the brain accounts for only approximately 2% of the bodyweight of a 70 kg adult, it consumes 20% of his or her total energy. The metabolic demand of the brain is met by blood flow that is protected at a high and privileged rate compared with other organs. Changes in brain glucose consumption also occur with age. Positron emission tomography (PET) has been used to chart brain metabolism (for example, using radiolabeled glucose or another metabolic substrate with a suitably short half-life).

The amount of glucose taken up by brain cells decreases with age. Sometimes these decreases can be linked to the development of mental symptoms or impairment such as memory decline. Consistent with the pattern of neuropathological lesions in Alzheimer's disease found at postmortem, regional cerebral metabolic studies in vivo show reduced glucose metabolism in the cortical association areas, with relative sparing of the subcortical structures and cerebellum. These reductions are greater the more severe the dementia. Similarly, longitudinal studies show that these changes in regional glucose metabolism precede and may predict later dementia onset.

Neurotransmitter changes. Levels of specific neurotransmitters decrease gradually with age. Most neurotransmitter systems show age-related decreases, and there are many indications that these decreases correspond with changes in cognitive function. The neurotransmitters involved with control of movement, attention, arousal, the sleep–wake cycle, eating and aggression are all found in discrete brain structures, and neurotransmitter loss caused by disease can often be related to the severity of symptoms associated with these structures.

This principle was first established for the neurotransmitter dopamine, which is lost in the substantia nigra (a region of the midbrain) of patients with Parkinson's disease. There is a widespread tendency towards loss of dopamine with normal aging, but in most individuals loss is moderate and without symptoms. In some cases, however, 90% or more of the dopaminergic neurons are lost and parkinsonian symptoms then appear. Similarly, loss of cells that release gamma-aminobutyric acid has been demonstrated in the caudate nucleus of patients with Huntington's disease. In Alzheimer's disease, there is a loss of cholinergic neurons projecting from the basal forebrain onto the cortex and hippocampus. Other age- and disease-related neurotransmitter abnormalities are shown in Table 2.1.

In general, clinical disease occurs only after extensive loss of neural integrity. This is in accordance with the concept of redundancy or 'brain reserve'. More specifically, the densities of receptors for neurotransmitters are critical determinants of the aging brain's capacity to respond to injury and to pharmaceutical agents.

TABLE 2.1

Age- and disease-related abnormalities in neurotransmitter systems

Transmitter/ enzyme	AD	HD	Alc	MID	PD	Aging
Ach-ChAT	↓↓↓	↓	↓	↔	↓	↓
AChE	↓↓	↓	↓	↔		↔
DA	↓	↓	↓		↓	↓
NE	↓		↓	↔		↓↓
GABA	↓	↓	↓			↓
5-HT	↓↓	↑			↓↓	↔
CRH	↓↓				↓	
SS	↓					↔
Glut	↓					↔

↓, decreased; ↑, increased; ↔, unchanged/uncertain.
Ach-ChAT, acetylcholine/choline acetyltransferase; AChE, acetylcholinesterase; AD, Alzheimer's disease; Alc, alcoholism; CRH, corticotropin-releasing hormone; DA, dopamine; GABA, gamma-aminobutyric acid; Glut, glutamate; HD, Huntington's disease; 5-HT, serotonin; MID, multi-infarct (vascular) dementia; NE, norepinephrine (noradrenaline); PD, Parkinson's disease; SS, somatostatin.

Microscopic changes with brain aging

Senile plaques are abnormal extracellular structures found in aging brains. They contain the debris of degenerating neurons, called neurites, embedded in an amorphous substance. Early investigators stained affected brain tissue sections and noted that this amorphous substance took up the dyes that stain plant starches, and so the structures were named 'amyloid' plaques (from the Latin *amylum* for starch). Later biochemical examination showed that this 'amyloid' material was composed mostly of a peptide fragment (variously termed Aβ or β-A4) that is cleaved from a large amyloid precursor protein (see Chapter 9). In the aging brain, senile plaques can be found at various stages of 'maturation', ranging from diffuse deposits of amyloid to the complex neuritic lesions typical of Alzheimer's disease (Figure 2.2).

Recent advances in brain imaging have detected amyloid fibrils in living animals and may soon be applied to humans. If sensitive and specific for Alzheimer's disease, these imaging techniques could make a huge contribution to the early diagnosis of dementing illnesses, long before major symptoms are provoked.

Amyloid is a novel substance, which the body's immune system may recognize as foreign. Not surprisingly, microglia (the small glial cells that function as the brain's 'scavengers') may be stimulated to intense metabolic activity in reaction to amyloid. In this process the glia consume oxygen and generate highly reactive oxygen-containing 'free radicals', as well as a host of pro-inflammatory or pro-oxidant chemical species called inflammatory cytokines. Detailed biochemical analysis of markers of microglial activation suggest that a low-grade inflammatory response occurs in the aging brain. Suppression of this response might explain why sustained use of non-steroidal anti-inflammatory drugs (NSAIDs) may retard the development of Alzheimer's disease (see Chapter 9).

Neurofibrillary tangles (NFTs, see Figure 2.2) are made up of abnormal aggregates of neurofilaments. Under the electron microscope these appear as pairs of 10 nm diameter filaments in the form of a double helix. The characteristically insoluble lesions probably originate as inclusions within the living neuronal cell body and are essentially

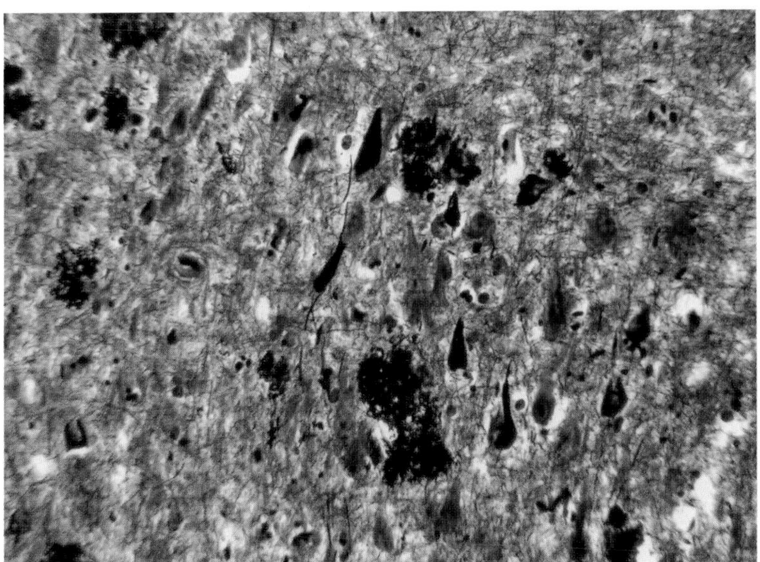

Figure 2.2 Brain tissue containing senile plaques and neurofibrillary tangles. (Von Braunmuhl stain). Image reproduced courtesy of Dr J Mackenzie, Aberdeen Royal Infirmary, UK.

biochemical modifications of the natural neuronal cytoskeleton. Although intraneuronal lesions by nature, NFTs are sometimes found between surviving neurons in patients with advanced Alzheimer's disease. These NFTs have been likened to 'ghosts' or 'gravestones' of their deceased cellular hosts.

NFTs are composed principally of altered forms of the naturally occurring microtubule-associated protein (MAP) called tau. Tau has several sites at which its composite amino acids may be substituted with a phosphate group. The tau in NFTs is hyperphosphorylated (i.e. it contains an abnormally large number of phosphate groups), making it more likely to aggregate into paired helical filaments. Tau proteins can also combine with glucose (glycation) as a result of oxidative stress linked to age-related abnormalities of glucose metabolism. Glycated tau can also promote the formation of paired helical filaments. When deposition of NFTs becomes extensive and involves the brain structures that are essential for memory, the symptoms of Alzheimer's disease are probably inevitable.

Selective cell loss in key brain structures

The key brain loci and structures that are important in brain aging are discussed below.

The hippocampi are bilateral structures critical to memory function. It was previously thought that brain cell loss in the hippocampi was the principal cause of memory impairment in 'normal' old age. However, we now know that the hippocampi do not lose brain cells as an inevitable consequence of aging. Instead, substantial hippocampal cell loss, when present, is a sign of neurodegenerative disease.

The frontal lobes play a role in the integration of cognitive and emotional responses to stimuli. It is here that diverse signals are integrated to support higher-order cognitive functions. The frontal lobes are strongly affected by aging, and there is now a consensus that several psychological changes (cognitive and functional decline) that occur with aging reflect deterioration of these structures. Like other cortical structures, the frontal lobes do not function symmetrically. Instead, one side is 'dominant' over the other.

Other structures. Some communicating subcortical frontal structures, and their corresponding dominant neurotransmitter systems, seem to be particularly vulnerable to aging. Normally aging humans, monkeys and rats show selective loss of cholinergic cells in the basal forebrain. This cholinergic deficit is closely related to the decline of memory function that is nearly universal in normal old people, but does not explain it in full. The dorsolateral prefrontal cortical regions are also vulnerable to age-related changes. These areas bear the distinction of having evolved last in the ontogeny of brain development, but it is not certain their changes with aging are related to this.

Functional changes with brain aging

Several of the common structural changes described above may be responsible for changes in mental abilities as people age, even though they may not be part of a dementing illness. Slowed mental processing is the most frequently detected age-related change in brain function.

Reaction time, which is a simple test of the time taken to respond to a defined stimulus, slows from early adulthood onwards. Most of this slowing occurs in the central nervous system rather than the peripheral nervous system, and it is most apparent in complex mental tasks.

Several mechanisms may account for mental slowing. Synaptic loss may slow information processing by depleting neuronal interconnections. Degradation of the myelin sheath in white-matter bundles may also slow information flow by decreasing the speed of signals in long bundles of axons. Such degradation is probably caused by age-related oxidation of fatty acids in the myelin by free radicals, via a process called membrane lipid peroxidation. Myelin peroxidation occurs in all brain cells from middle age onwards. These changes in white matter are detectable using diffusion tensor imaging (see page 21). Similar oxidative changes may also affect the large regulatory biomolecules in neuronal membranes.

'Successful' aging

While common changes relating to brain aging are typically deleterious to cognitive and functional abilities, an increasing proportion of old people avoid significant loss in these abilities. This trend is one of the notable successes of modern geriatric medicine, and in some instances it challenges our concepts of 'normal' brain aging. Although mild-to-moderate degrees of cognitive decline were previously attributed simply to 'old age', this idea is no longer tenable.

One explanation for the 'successful aging' phenomenon is to question whether the usual above-described functional changes are in fact a subtle manifestation of one or more neurodegenerative processes that are common – but not ubiquitous – in old age. If these changes were simply part of aging, the implication would be that all people (or nearly all) would develop clinical symptoms if they lived long enough. The fact that some elderly people do 'age successfully' negates the idea of cognitive decline as part of 'normal brain aging'. Instead, the decline appears to result from mild pathological conditions that are extremely prevalent, but not ubiquitous, in old age.

Another explanation is that the neurocognitive or functional changes that typically accompany aging may appear only when a vulnerable or aged brain is required to function in a setting of poor general physical health. This sort of decline in physical health is increasingly avoidable and disease-free elderly people often show less decline in cognitive abilities than was commonly considered the norm for their age. 'Successful aging' individuals therefore demonstrate the importance of maintaining general health for preservation of cognitive as well as physical functioning. Table 2.2 lists a number of common medical conditions that can impair cognition in the elderly and are therefore appropriate targets for intervention in the interests of maintaining cognitive abilities into old age.

TABLE 2.2

Medical conditions that can impair cognition in old age

Common	Rare
• Infection – bronchopneumonia – urinary tract infection • Cardiorespiratory – myocardial infarction – congestive heart failure – atrial fibrillation • Nutritional – vitamin deficiency • Endocrine – hypothyroidism – hypocalcemia – diabetes mellitus • Neoplasia – most tumors	• Inflammatory – sarcoidosis – systemic lupus erythematosus • Metabolic disorders • Trauma – subdural hematoma

Key points – the aging brain

- In the absence of dementia, brain shrinkage is normal after 50 years of age. It is largely explained by reduced brain cell size, not by brain cell death.
- Clinical severity of dementia symptoms is related to loss of neurotransmitters, especially acetylcholine.
- Senile ('amyloid') plaques are present with aging in the absence of dementia. Neurofibrillary tangles and loss of synaptic density are more strongly associated with dementia.
- With aging there is mental slowing, attributable to reduced synaptic efficiency and degradation of information-transfer systems inside the brain.
- Age-related changes in the frontal cortex probably explain most cognitive impairment with aging in the absence of dementia.

Key references

Barger SW, Harmon AD. Microglial activation by Alzheimer amyloid precursor protein and modulation by apolipoprotein E. *Nature* 1997;388: 878–81.

Bohr VA, Ottersen OP, Tønjum T. Genome instability and DNA repair in brain, ageing and neurological disease. *Neuroscience* 2007; 145:1183–6.

Braak H, Braak E. Evolution of neuronal changes in the course of Alzheimer's disease. *J Neural Transmission* 1998;53(suppl): 127–40.

Finch CE. The biology of aging in model organisms. *Alzheimer Dis Assoc Disord* 2003;17(suppl 2): S39–41.

Flood DG, Coleman PD. Neuron numbers and sizes in aging brain – comparisons of human, monkey and rodent data. *Neurobiol Aging* 1988;9:453–63.

Green MS, Kaye JA, Ball MJ. The Oregon brain ageing study: neuropathology accompanying healthy ageing in the oldest old. *Neurology* 2000;54:105–13.

Martin GM. The genetics and epigenetics of altered proliferative homeostasis in ageing and cancer. *Mech Ageing Dev* 2007;128:9–12.

Martin JE, Sheaff MT. The pathology of ageing: concepts and mechanisms. *J Pathol* 2007;211:111–13.

Moreira PI, Smith MA, Zhu X et al. Oxidative stress and neurodegeneration. *Ann NY Acad Sci* 2005;1043:545–52.

Mouton PR, Martin LJ, Calhoun ME et al. Cognitive decline strongly correlates with cortical atrophy in Alzheimer's dementia. *Neurobiol Aging* 1998;19:371–7.

Perry G, Raina AK, Nunomura A et al. How important is oxidative damage? Lessons from Alzheimer's disease. *Free Radic Biol Med* 2000; 28:831–4.

Peters R. Ageing and the brain. *Postgrad Med J* 2006;82:84–8.

Riga D, Riga S, Halalau F, Schneider F. Brain lipopigment accumulation in normal and pathological aging. *Ann N Y Acad Sci* 2006;1067:158-63.

Schmitt FA, Davis DG, Wekstein DR et al. "Preclinical" AD revisited: neuropathology of cognitively normal older adults. *Neurology* 2000;55:370–6.

Toescu EC. Normal brain ageing: models and mechanisms. *Philos Trans R Soc Lond B Biol Sci* 2005; 360:2347–54.

3 Symptoms, signs and course

Neurodegenerative brain changes at the molecular, subcellular, cellular or tissue levels can reach a threshold level of severity at which cognitive capacities are lost. Some neurodegenerative conditions such as Alzheimer's and Parkinson's diseases may represent exaggerations of 'normal' aging processes (see previous chapter), but many certainly do not. Certain broad principles that apply are described below.

The 'threshold–decompensation' model

The 'threshold–decompensation' model of symptom formation that applies to many organ systems can also be applied to cognitive decline, as illustrated in Figure 3.1. Cognitive capacities normally grow through infancy and childhood so that optimal functional capacity is attained in early adulthood (left-hand, ascending portion of curve). The measure of this optimum cognitive capacity may be influenced by genes and also by

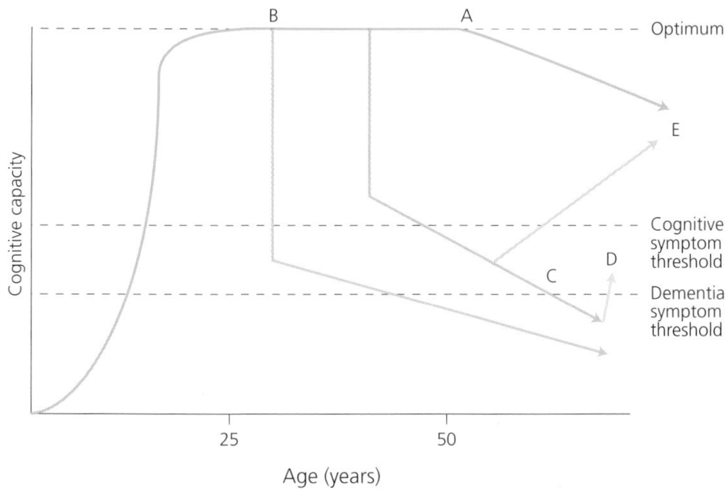

Figure 3.1 Trajectories of cognitive development and decline (see text for explanation).

childhood illnesses, education, nutrition or exposure to neurotoxins. Exposure to severe harmful influences may limit brain development so that optimum functional maturity is not attained, as is seen in neurodevelopmental disorders. Upon attaining optimum development, the 'normal' cognitive capacity curve typically begins to decline slowly, several decades after reaching its optimum, at about 50 years of age (point A in Figure 3.1). However, a catastrophic event (point B) such as a traumatic brain injury or stroke can suddenly disrupt brain integrity or function beyond the critical symptom threshold, below which cognitive symptoms appear. Such injury can result in cognitive disability. Other injuries may be insufficient to cause an observable cognitive syndrome but nonetheless may reduce the brain's cognitive reserve so that the 'normal' aging trajectory now proceeds from a lower starting point (green line). Accelerated decline in the trajectory now crosses the symptom threshold in relatively early old age (point C). In some instances, functional integrity may be re-established with treatment of (or recovery from) the insult, leading to a partial recovery (point D) or complete restitution of capacities (point E). Then, the age when obvious cognitive symptoms appear is affected minimally, if at all.

Cognitive disorders: delirium, dementia and focal syndromes

Insults that cause disarray in the functional capacity of the brain may result in different cognitive syndromes.

- Fulminant neurodegenerative processes (rarely) or severe alterations of the brain's metabolic milieu (more commonly) can provoke delirium.
- Slow neurodegenerative processes or more chronic injury states typically provoke dementia.
- Focal neurological injuries may provoke monofocal cognitive deficits.

Although these syndromes share the cardinal feature of cognitive decline, they are otherwise distinct.

Delirium. The hallmark of delirium is clouding of consciousness. Other common features include abnormalities of emotion, perception and behavior, as well as cognition. The terms 'delirium' and 'confusion' are sometimes used interchangeably when clouding of consciousness produces changes in mental capacities. The term 'delirium' has a more precise meaning than 'confusion' and is therefore preferred.

Two important aspects of consciousness are:

- the level of arousal (from coma to stupor to normal vigilance and beyond)
- the ability to alter or focus one's attention at will and to discriminate between several simultaneous environmental stimuli.

In delirium, an individual with a relatively normal state of arousal may still have reduced ability to perceive and distinguish between competing stimuli. The result is a reduced capacity to focus attention on a task at hand, to sustain that attention, or to move it at will to another task. Abnormal visual phenomena are also common and may include misinterpretation of visual stimuli (illusions) or visual perception in the absence of an appropriate stimulus (hallucinations).

Delirium usually develops over a period of hours, tends to fluctuate in severity, and may be interspersed with periods of normality. A delirious patient's world is often colored by emotional responses to distorted experiences. Intense fear or panic may result from bizarre or threatening visual hallucinations. Such visual symptoms, the characteristic fluctuating course and the patient's preoccupation with his/her own inner world are useful clues to the presence of delirium.

Delirium is often provoked by an abnormality in the metabolic substrate required for normal brain function. The clinician's task is therefore to identify the provoking cause such as poisoning or electrolyte imbalance. When identified, such causes are often reversible, and successful treatment usually results in symptomatic improvement. However, delirium can be among the most vexing of all conditions to treat. Often, despite diligent efforts, the provoking toxic or metabolic derangement cannot be identified and therefore cannot be directly treated. In this case, conservative and supportive care must be offered in the hope that the condition will resolve spontaneously.

Delirium has a complex relationship with the types of chronic progressive brain disease that typically provoke dementia. Chronic brain disease does not usually provoke alteration in consciousness. Thus, the course of neurodegenerative disease may not include delirious states, but their resultant compromise to brain integrity can nonetheless promote vulnerability to a delirium provoked by an additional insult. Thus, physically healthy people with clinically inapparent pre-existing brain disease may be more vulnerable to the development of delirium when they become physically ill. When the pre-existing brain disease is severe enough to have provoked dementia, an added insult may result in delirium that is superimposed on dementia. The resulting clinical picture may be perplexing.

Thus, a new or unexpected occurrence of delirium may be an early indicator of a neurodegenerative disease or may also signal the presence of a severe but previously unsuspected medical illness. The case-fatality rate with delirium is substantial (though much improved with modern care); the appearance of delirium is therefore a warning sign that requires immediate attention. Upon recovery from delirium, patients with pre-existing dementia will typically revert to a clinical appearance of uncomplicated dementia.

Dementia. Sometimes, particularly in the UK, the term 'dementia' is used to signify a brain disease with a precise corresponding neuropathology. However, we prefer to define dementia as a *clinical syndrome* without implication of any specific etiology. The syndrome is characterized by a decline in multiple aspects of cognition that is not attributable to alteration in consciousness. Dementia symptoms may include impairment in:

- memory
- reasoning
- language
- perceptual interpretation
- ability to deal with visuospatial relationships
- personal judgment
- 'praxis', the usually extra-conscious ability to order and coordinate movements or activities to achieve some simple goals such as walking or writing
- 'gnostic' functions, the ability (usually taken for granted) to interpret cognitively what is adequately perceived in any of the five primary sensory modalities.

Neuropsychiatric classification systems. There are two standard classification systems for dementia: the American Psychiatric Association's *Diagnostic and Statistical Manual of Mental Disorders*, currently in its fourth edition (DSM-IV), and the tenth revision of the World Health Organization's *International Statistical Classification of Diseases and Related Health Problems* (ICD-10). Both systems use broad definitions of dementia but apply somewhat different operational terms. Both require a decline in memory and other abilities to a degree that interferes with everyday activities. The ICD-10 also requires alteration in personality, while DSM-IV specifically notes apraxia, aphasia (loss of language abilities), agnosia (e.g. failure to recognize a familiar face) and problems in executive functioning (planning, organizing, sequencing, abstracting) as other areas of deficit. The DSM-IV criteria for dementia of the Alzheimer's type are given in Table 3.1. Both classification systems regard memory loss as necessary for a diagnosis of dementia; however, some illnesses – notably frontotemporal lobe dementia (see below) – occur commonly without much memory difficulty, at least in their early stages. Future revisions of both sets of criteria will therefore need to deal with this issue.

Dementia is sometimes taken to imply irreversibility, and it is true that most dementing illnesses are incurable. However, irreversibility is not a defining feature. A number of specific causes of dementia provoke a fully or at least partially recoverable state (Table 3.2). Indeed, a thorough search for the cause(s) of dementia, including specifically reversible causes, is essential.

Dementia following stroke. Stroke is the third most common cause of death and the most common cause of chronic disability. An acute stroke consists of a core of dead brain cells surrounded by an ischemic penumbra ('shadow') in the brain where cells are alive but are not functioning effectively. The penumbra contributes to acute clinical deficits at first and then, if the blood supply does not return to normal, to the chronic deficits. In the post-stroke period, recovery typically takes weeks or months but can vary substantially even between patients with apparently identical structural damage. The source of these individual differences is unknown. Recovery processes after a stroke depend on innate reconstructive processes that stimulate brain

TABLE 3.1

Diagnostic criteria for dementia of the Alzheimer's type based on DSM-IV

A.* The development of multiple cognitive deficits manifested by:

(1) memory impairment (impaired ability to learn new information or to recall previously learned information)

AND

(2) one (or more) of the following cognitive disturbances:

(a) aphasia (language disturbance)

(b) apraxia (impaired ability to carry out motor activities despite intact motor function)

(c) agnosia (failure to recognize or identify objects despite intact sensory function)

(d) disturbance in executive function (i.e. planning, organizing, sequencing, abstracting)

B. The cognitive deficits in criteria A1 and A2 each cause significant impairment in social or occupational functioning and represent a significant decline from a previous level of functioning

C.† The course is characterized by gradual onset and continuing cognitive decline

D. The cognitive deficits in criteria A1 and A2 are not due to any of the following:

(1) other central nervous system conditions that cause progressive deficits in memory and cognition (e.g. cerebrovascular disease, Parkinson's disease, Huntington's disease, subdural hematoma, normal-pressure hydrocephalus, brain tumor)

(2) systemic conditions that are known to cause dementia (e.g. hypothyroidism, vitamin B_{12} or folic acid deficiency, niacin deficiency, hypercalcemia, neurosyphilis, HIV infection

(3) substance-induced conditions

E. The deficits do not occur exclusively during the course of a delirium

F. The disturbance is not better accounted for by another Axis 1 disorder (e.g. major depressive disorder, schizophrenia)

CONTINUED

TABLE 3.1 (CONTINUED)

*This section describes the criteria for dementia that are specified in the DSM-IV for each of many different dementing illnesses and are therefore identified commonly as 'DSM-IV criteria for dementia'. There is controversy about the absolute requirement of memory impairment, which can be lacking or subtle in some dementing illnesses such as frontotemporal lobe dementia.
†Some experts dispute the requirement that dementia must have an insidious onset (e.g. some stroke patients have sudden onset of dementia), or the notion that dementia must necessarily be progressive (e.g. some patients with traumatic brain injury may be left with a dementia syndrome that is stable and not progressive).
DSM-IV, *Diagnostic and Statistical Manual of Mental Disorders*, 4th edn. American Psychiatric Association, 2000.

TABLE 3.2

Specific causes of dementia that provoke a fully or partially recoverable state

Cause	Treatment
Depressive illness	Antidepressants, electroconvulsive therapy, psychotherapy
Drug intoxication	Discontinuation of the offending agent, supportive therapy, specific antidotes occasionally
Normal-pressure hydrocephalus	Surgical shunt
Infectious illness	Antibiotics
Neoplasia	Steroids for any associated edema
Cardiovascular disease	Specific therapy to correct hypertension, ischemia, etc.
Subdural hematoma	Surgical evacuation
Metabolic/endocrine	Specific corrective therapy

remodeling; these appear to act synergistically with rehabilitative measures and may involve the recruitment of neural networks and pathways not previously used (see 'Synaptic plasticity' page 17). Cognitive deficits conform to these patterns; some are dense and unremitting, others improve slowly and some seem to be initiated by the acute stroke and to evolve gradually to appear indistinguishable from Alzheimer's disease.

Focal cerebral disorders. In contrast with dementia, focal disorders are specific or limited to functional impairment in one or, at most, two domains of cognitive ability. Although they are sometimes associated with large strokes, focal syndromes more often result from more circumscribed brain injury. Affected cognitive domains may include language (aphasia) or interpretation of perception (agnosia). Because they do not produce a global decline in cognition, these conditions do not qualify as dementia. Instead, the typical psychological symptoms linked to various regions of the brain may be conveniently divided between the frontal lobes, parietal lobes, temporal lobes and occipital lobes (Table 3.3).

Frontal lobe lesions produce some of the most perplexing symptoms of focal cerebral disease. Frontal lobe dysfunction can produce either an apathetic state or an opposite disinhibition with over-expansive behaviors, social intrusiveness and loss of social and moral control. Such patients can show errors of judgment in almost any field of human endeavor. Sometimes they may also show an empty or fatuous cheerfulness without meaning or significance. The ability to maintain attention or carry out sequential planned activities (executive functioning) is often affected.

Parietal lobe lesions (of either parietal lobe) typically cause visuospatial and topographical difficulties or agnosia. Visuospatial problems may be detected during clinical examination by asking the patient to produce or copy simple drawings, such as a cube or clock face, or to construct simple patterns from matchsticks. Topographical problems become apparent when the patient has difficulty in negotiating a new environment, for example being unable to find the way out, or getting lost or stranded in familiar surroundings. When the dominant parietal lobe is affected, complex language defects may also appear, including alexia (inability to read) and agraphia (inability to write). Motor coordination and praxis are often disturbed. Non-dominant parietal lobe lesions disturb awareness of body image and its relation to external space. Degenerative changes to the parietal lobe in dementing illnesses (typical of middle- or late-stage Alzheimer's disease) can cause dressing apraxia (inability to conceptualize or execute the routine task of putting on clothes in

TABLE 3.3
Functions subject to localized cortical impairment

Frontal lobe
- Responsiveness and involvement (apathy)
- Response inhibition ('disinhibition')
- Movement planning
- Task sequencing, planning and organization

Parietal lobe
- Somatosensory integration
- Tactile form recognition
- Visual perception
- Spatial relations
- Language (mostly receptive and interpretive)
- Praxis
- Motor coordination

Temporal lobe
- Auditory processing
- Visual processing
- Verbal memory
- Language (mostly expressive)

Occipital lobe
- Visual recognition

the correct orientation or in appropriate order) and various forms of agnosia.

Temporal lobe lesions. The temporal lobes contain the hippocampi, and the dominant temporal lobe is closely associated with language abilities. Thus, temporal lobe lesions cause problems with memory and language. The latter may include both expressive and sensory difficulties (the inability to create language or interpret it). Lesions of the non-dominant temporal lobes tend to show fewer signs or symptoms. It is worth noting that severe memory loss does not occur with lesions of one temporal lobe alone – bilateral injury is required to produce amnesia.

Lesions in anterior temporal lobe structures such as the amygdalae can cause persistent disturbances in temperament and the control of aggressive impulses. Unlike other focal brain lesions, injuries to the temporal lobe that extend deep into its structure can produce a characteristic visual-field defect. This is caused by damage to the temporal radiation of axons that convey visual information from the lateral geniculate body in the brainstem to the occipital lobes. Neurodegenerative dementing illnesses do not typically cause such damage. Because these axonal tracts carry visual information (from both eyes) from only the right or left side of a person's visual field, this sort of visual-field defect indicates a focal temporal lobe brain lesion, for example from trauma, a tumor or stroke.

Occipital lobe lesions. All of the symptoms of occipital lobe lesions are linked in some way to visual functions. Symptoms range from 'cortical blindness' to a less dramatic inability to read while retaining the ability to write (alexia without agraphia), or failure to identify colors or objects. The occipital lobes are not usually involved in neurodegenerative dementing illnesses.

Personality changes

As with cognitive capacities, personality may change as a person ages, either as a result of 'normal' developmental processes or as a reflection of brain disease. In healthy aging, personality traits are usually quite stable with the exception that some elderly people become more preoccupied with their own mental life. If there is a stereotypical personality change with aging, it is decreased impulsivity, fear of sudden change and preoccupation with orderliness. These features of 'normal' aging may be exaggerated by longer life expectancy among inflexible, stronger personality types, causing over-representation of this type among the very old. If personality changes deviate from the above, or are out of keeping with earlier traits, it is likely that such changes reflect an underlying brain disease. Indeed, personality change can sometimes herald the later emergence of a frank dementia syndrome.

Key points – symptoms, signs and course

- The cerebral reserve hypothesis proposes that brain disease or damage must exceed a reserve of cerebral ('cognitive') capacities before cognitive symptoms are detectable.
- Delirium is characterized by clouding of consciousness and corresponding disturbances of emotion, perception and behavior. It tends to fluctuate in severity and may be interspersed with episodes of normality. It is often reversible, but complex associations with chronic progressive brain disease are common.
- Dementia is the clinical syndrome of global cognitive decline that is not attributable to a disturbance of consciousness.
- Reversible ('treatable') causes of dementia must be evaluated in the early investigation of cognitive impairment in old people.
- Localized cortical impairment is often associated with specific cognitive deficits related to the specific functions of the area of impaired cortex (e.g. parietal lobe damage is linked to visuospatial deficits) and may not otherwise provoke dementia.

Key references

Jacoby R, Oppenheimer C, Dening T, Thomas A, eds. *Oxford Textbook of Old Age Psychiatry*, 4th edn. Oxford: Oxford University Press, 2008.

Light LL, Burke DM. *Language, Memory, and Aging*. Cambridge: Cambridge University Press, 1988.

Lishman WA. *Organic Psychiatry: The Psychological Consequences of Cerebral Disorder*, 3rd edn. Oxford: Blackwell Science, 1997.

Rabins PV, Lyketsos CG, Steele CD. *Practical Dementia Care*, 2nd edn. New York: Oxford University Press, 2006.

Ropper AH, Brown RH. *Adams and Victor's Principles of Neurology*, 8th edn. Baltimore: McGraw-Hill, 2005.

4 Neuropsychiatric complications

Although the neurodegenerative diseases that cause dementia characteristically attack brain structures that are essential for cognition, their effects are not limited to these regions. Other affected areas of the brain may include those responsible for mood or emotional responsivity, or for regulation of arousal-modifying neurotransmitters such as dopamine or norepinephrine (noradrenaline). When these regions are diseased, patients with dementia commonly develop non-cognitive symptoms such as hallucinations and delusions, pervasive disturbances of mood or various troublesome behavioral anomalies.

Generally, these symptoms may be categorized using terms familiar to psychiatrists for the description of psychopathology in other mental illnesses. Such symptoms usually cause considerable distress to patients and especially to their carers, to the point that they can e decisive determinants of the need for placement or other urgent intervention.

Delusions and hallucinations

Delusions. A delusion is an unshakable belief that is implausible, idiosyncratic and wholly embraced by the patient. Delusional beliefs are common in dementing illness, where their fixed quality and pervasive nature are often revealed by the patient's recurrent behavior.

Typical delusions in dementia include the idea that one's home is not one's own, or that a spouse or carer has been replaced by a stranger. Sometimes, the delusion appears to serve the purpose of making good or explaining a deficit in memory; for example, mislaid or forgotten household items may become the subject of delusional beliefs that a thief has entered the home and taken the items. Even if someone else later locates the 'stolen' item, the demented patient often remains unconvinced and may remark on how cunning the 'thief' was to replace the item before his capture.

Hallucinations are sensory perceptions that occur without adequate stimulus and can occur in any of the five primary sensory modalities.

Visual hallucinations are common in delirium but rare in most other psychiatric conditions. Visual phenomena can be encountered at any point during the course of a dementing illness. These visual disturbances are usually fleeting and do not exactly meet formal definitions of hallucinations even though they are conveniently referred to as such. They occur fairly often in dementia, and are especially characteristic of Lewy body dementia (see next chapter) in which they may have an illusory quality, being triggered by otherwise neutral stimuli such as the television, a wallpaper pattern or a crumpled bed sheet. Often they are part of complex hallucinatory phenomena involving several senses, for example both vision and hearing.

By themselves these experiences have little diagnostic importance, but they can become a source of great distress, especially when other family members are perceived, sometimes long after their death. The content of hallucination in dementia is often threatening or perplexing to the patient, provoking agitated or troublesome behavior. Persistent or recurrent hallucinations of a single form may also engender secondary delusional beliefs; for example, repeated visions of a deceased spouse may lead the sufferer to believe that the spouse is still alive. In these circumstances, the emotional reaction to the false perception requires comfort and reassurance.

Mood abnormalities

Dementing illnesses sometimes first appear with clinical symptoms of depression, and depressed mood is a common feature of lzheimer's disease and several other common neurodegenerative diseases, including Parkinson's disease and stroke. Patients with insight may feel sad or despondent about their loss of cognitive abilities, although this reaction is less common than might be imagined. More common are depressive changes that are typical of 'major depression', such as psychomotor slowing or apathy, disturbed sleep and appetite, self-neglect or self-reproach, and nihilistic ideas of impoverishment or physical illness.

The common co-occurrence of dementia syndromes and clinical depression can occasionally create diagnostic challenges; however, depressive features should be treated regardless of whether they are secondary to a neurodegenerative disorder.

Case report 1

Mrs H, aged 82, was visited by a nurse at home. Her daughter who lived a few houses away was also present. Mrs H complained that men had entered her home and taken things during the previous few months. Items 'stolen' included mementoes from her husband, a photograph album and a broken antique clock. In fact, she said, she had caught the men only the other night and that the police had come and arrested them. Her daughter explained that her mother had simply 'mislaid' some of the items (they were all easily found by her grandson) and that the clock had been sent for repair. The alleged episode with the men and police reflected events of a few nights previously when Mrs H had walked to her daughter's house in an agitated state, stating that men were fighting in her living room and that the police were there. The grandson noted that this account fitted events in a police program currently showing on the television. 'Mom', said the daughter, 'it was the television you were watching. A police story. Now, don't worry. Just sit down, and have you remembered to lock up and bring your keys?' The mother replied that she had, and handed her daughter the remote control for the television.

Comment: Delusions of theft are common in dementia. Typically, the delusions account for an object that has been mislaid and the person with dementia has forgotten where it might be. Without a search strategy, the loss of the objects is 'explained' by theft.

Other patients with dementia may show agitation, excessive worry or arousal, or exaggerated fears. All of these mood states may motivate a variety of untoward or troublesome behaviors that can substantially increase the burden or complexity of care.

Behavioral disturbances

Behavioral anomalies in dementia can be conveniently divided into new and unwanted behaviors, or the loss or neglect of normal and desired behaviors. New behaviors can often be attributed to the presence of hallucinations or delusions. Similarly, aggression and irritability can sometimes be linked to abnormal persecutory ideas. By contrast, some repetitive or stereotyped behaviors can be traced to over-learned or overrehearsed occupational or domestic tasks. A severely demented mailman, for example, may wander a regular route around his residential home mailing pieces of newspaper into unlikely crevices. Typically, it is the new behaviors, which derive from psychosis or altered perception of reality, that are most likely to improve with carefully monitored pharmacotherapy.

Sometimes the disappearance of old behaviors can be even more distressing to family or friends. Deficits can extend across a wide range of activities including dressing, use of sanitary facilities and eating. As dementia progresses, carers can become surprisingly resourceful in developing compensatory strategies. Self-care routines, though tiresome for a daughter with a demented mother, can sometimes become playful or even humorous. While such 'comic relief' may leaven the day, one must never forget the seriousness of the deficit, which may pose a constant hazard to the health and safety of the patient and others.

Case report 2

Mrs B was a 74-year-old who had been widowed 2 years previously. Recently, her neighbors had become concerned by her leaving the apartment block at about 2 AM to go 'shopping for my husband's dinner'. At home assessment she had many features of dementia. Her routine included repeatedly cleaning and pressing her husband's old clothes, preparing meals for him and identifying to observers where she saw him in the room. Unusually, she had placed a framed photograph of him at his place at the dining table. The cover glass had been removed from the photograph and the area around his mouth was worn thin by her kissing and trying to press food through an aperture she had made.

Comment: Disorientation in time is common. The person with dementia is unable to to identify the temporal and social clues that keep him/her in step with daily activities. Forgetting that a loved husband is dead, the widow continues to nurture his memory and takes comfort from following her routine. Although the actions may seem bizarre, when considered together they can be seen as measures that sustain a sense of continuity with the past and deny the despair that full acceptance of death would cause.

Key points – neuropsychiatric complications

- Neuropsychiatric complications are extremely prevalent in dementia, and can be important determinants of the ability of individuals with dementia to live with only minimal to moderate assistance.
- Low or irritable mood may occur at any stage of dementia but often responds to antidepressant treatment. The diagnosis of depressive disorder in a person with dementia may be complicated by coexistent symptoms of the dementia itself, such as disturbance of language or perception.
- Delusions and hallucinations are also frequent in dementia. When compelling, they can be among the most troublesome neuropsychiatric complications, necessitating close management.
- Behavioral disturbances in dementia may be grouped into new unwanted behaviors (e.g. aggression) and failure to perform desired behaviors (e.g. loss of domestic skills).
- Patients with dementia also fall into three broad clusters depending on their neuropsychiatric or behavioral symptoms. These symptoms, when present, seem to cluster into affective and psychotic groupings.

Epidemiology

Recent longitudinal population studies have examined the rates of neuropsychiatric complications in community-based cohorts of patients with dementia. The findings show that these complications are highly prevalent in those diagnosed with dementia, at least half of whom are reported to have one or more neuropsychiatric or behavioral symptoms. Furthermore, among those who are initially without such symptoms, at least half appear to develop one or more new symptoms over the subsequent 18 months.

Classification

A recent empirical analysis of neuropsychiatric symptoms in dementia suggests that the patients fall into three broad groups with different patterns of neuropsychiatric symptoms.

- At any one time, almost half of patients have no such symptoms, or one at most (asymptomatic cluster).
- A similar number have two or more symptoms that are in the realm of mood, arousal, irritability, activity level and the like (affective cluster).
- Finally, a small group of patients experience hallucinations or delusions of sufficient intensity or frequency to have a major bearing on their or their carer's quality of life (psychotic cluster).

As we learn more about neuropsychiatric complications of dementia and their treatment, it may be useful to rely increasingly on this categorical framework.

Key references

Cumming JL, Mega MS. *Neuropsychiatry and Behavioral Neuroscience*. New York: Oxford University Press, 2003.

Lyketsos CG, Steinberg M, Tschanz JT et al. Mental and behavioral disturbances in dementia: findings from the Cache County Study on Memory in Aging. *Am J Psychiatry* 2000;157:708–14.

Meeks TW, Ropacki SA, Jeste DV. The neurobiology of neuropsychiatric syndromes in dementia. *Curr Opin Psychiatry* 2006;19:581–6.

Onyike CU, Sheppard JM, Tschanz JT et al. Epidemiology of apathy in older adults: the Cache County Study. *Am J Geriatr Psychiatry* 2007;15:365–75.

Rabins PV, Lyketsos CG, Steele CD. *Practical Dementia Care*, 2nd edn. New York: Oxford University Press, 2006.

5 Clinical examination and investigations

Differential diagnosis of dementia

Once it is established that a patient has a dementia syndrome, the clinician's task is to identify the underlying brain pathology. In general, severity of dementia cannot be simply equated to the extent and nature of brain pathology because other disease-modifying factors seem to be at work. That said, certain characteristics lead to a differential diagnosis, which is often helpful for the evaluation of prognosis and methods of treatment. Because Alzheimer's disease is by far the most common cause of dementia, we discuss it first. The clinical diagnosis of Alzheimer's dementia is established in three ways.

First, what is the age of the patient? The incidence of Alzheimer's disease doubles with each 5 years of age (which exceeds the age-related increase of other causes of dementia); thus, in general, the older the patient, the more likely the diagnosis of Alzheimer's disease (see also Chapter 8).

Second, one looks for signs or symptoms that suggest other causes of dementia. Alzheimer's disease then becomes a diagnosis of exclusion. The process begins with laboratory evaluation of reversible causes. Other brain disorders can often accompany the development of Alzheimer neuropathology but:

- such pathology in itself does not produce *focal motor neurological changes* (which are more typical of vascular dementia)
- it is not typically associated with *sudden stepwise decrements in function* (as is sometimes true of vascular dementia)
- usually there are no *associated symptoms of Parkinson's disease* (although some hypertonicity and cogwheel tremor may be evident in patients with moderately advanced disease)
- it does not typically present with *predominant language or behavior changes in the absence of memory difficulty* (as is sometimes true of frontotemporal dementia)
- it does not present with *fulminant symptoms or myoclonus* (as is more typical of prion diseases).

Another distinction is sometimes made when the patient presents with rigidity, fluctuation in consciousness and prominent visual hallucinosis, which are typical of Lewy body dementia. Beyond this, one should also attempt to exclude other rarer causes of dementia such as Huntington's disease (choreo-athetosis and family history), progressive supranuclear palsy or Wernicke's encephalopathy (ophthalmoplegias), or hydrocephalus (gait difficulties with urinary incontinence).

When these rarer causes of dementia are not suspected, the diagnosis of Alzheimer's disease can be made more secure by observation of certain cognitive and functional symptoms and signs that are typical of the disease and therefore tend to confirm the diagnosis. Prominent among these is a clinical course that begins with memory difficulty but spreads to involve language functions, praxis or gnostic dysfunction. Often these latter changes are subtly present *before* the patient has unambiguous dementia, in which instance they create a clinical impression that the patient is in a prodromal phase of Alzheimer's disease. Even if these subtle changes cannot be identified, patients are sometimes noted to have functional difficulties that cannot be explained by deficits in memory alone – a picture that is again suggestive of mild or prodromal Alzheimer's disease.

A stepwise plan to establishing the diagnosis

Accurate diagnosis provides the basis for good clinical practice. Because information of many sorts may be considered in the diagnostic process, we recommend that the examining clinician collects and organizes clinical information using a purpose-designed template that can be completed easily, follows logical steps, and is easy to check and summarize. The steps in the following summary are explained more fully below.

- Step 1 is a full medical history, which usually involves an informant.
- Step 2 is a full physical, neurological and laboratory examination, focusing on findings that can contribute to differential diagnosis (see above).
- Step 3 is a comprehensive mental status and cognitive evaluation. This is useful for clinical characterization of the dementia syndrome

and establishes a baseline level of ability that can serve as a guide and measure of progressive dementia.

- Step 4 assesses behavioral and neuropsychiatric symptoms of dementia. While these symptoms may sometimes trigger referral, they are often not raised at examination until asked about directly.
- Step 5 addresses functional capacity to complete everyday tasks.
- Step 6 involves the use of diagnostic imaging, to identify either unsuspected lesions such as frontal tumors or old 'silent' strokes, or for the evaluation of contributing cerebrovascular disease.
- Step 7 is optional, and involves referral for specialized diagnostic investigation such as imaging procedures that are typically available only in specialty clinics and research centers, or collection of cerebrospinal fluid for analysis of Alzheimer's disease biomarkers.

Step 1: medical history. The most important part of any clinical evaluation is the history, which is usually obtained from the carer or another well-informed third party. The examiner must first seek and document evidence that the patient's present state represents *a decline* from a prior level of abilities. The natural history of the illness (prodrome, onset, course, prominent symptoms) is then recorded. Was disease onset insidious – as is usual in Alzheimer's disease – or sudden, as in a stroke? Did symptoms progress smoothly and inexorably, typical of Alzheimer's disease, or in a pattern of stepwise decline, which suggests a vascular process? Specific symptoms may have differential diagnostic significance. For example, if the patient has been ill for several years, has he or she developed the prominent difficulties with language, praxis or gnostic functions that are typical of Alzheimer's disease? The medical history can be equally informative. Are there risk factors for cerebrovascular illness, such as diabetes, atrial fibrillation, poorly controlled hypertension or generalized atherosclerosis? Is there a history of alcohol misuse or exposure to other toxins?

Step 2: physical, neurological and laboratory examination are nearly as important. Perhaps 5% of old people with apparent dementia have an underlying physical illness that, when treated, effectively improves their mental function (see Table 3.2, page 37). Most of these conditions are revealed, at least in part, by careful physical examination, and the physical findings can be enhanced by routine laboratory tests. A complete physical and neurological examination is therefore essential. The following tests should be performed routinely:

- measurement of blood pressure
- auscultation for carotid bruits
- chest auscultation
- hematology, including differential cell count and erythrocyte sedimentation rate (optional)
- biochemistry (glucose and electrolytes, calcium and phosphate, thyroid function tests and simple urinalysis) and hepatic function tests (alanine aminotransferase, serum albumin) as well as renal clearance tests (measurement of creatinine and blood urea nitrogen is inexpensive and useful).

As the relationship between dementia and glucose tolerance becomes better understood, assessment of glycated hemoglobin (HbA_{1c}) may also become a routine procedure in the diagnosis of dementia. Although vitamin deficiencies are a rare cause of dementia in the developed world, measurements of vitamin B_{12}, folate and homocysteine are inexpensive and are recommended. Rarely, tests for HIV, syphilis, Borrelia, and Lyme titer will be informative. Routine cerebrospinal fluid examination is not recommended.

The neurological examination need not be overly complex. Are extra-occular movements intact? Do focal motor or reflex changes show asymmetry, suggesting stroke or tumor? Are there features of Parkinson's disease, such as slowed movements and mentation, tremor, difficulties with phonation or gait disturbance? Have these responded to treatment, for example with L-dopa? Gait should be checked for apraxia (the patient appears to be effortfully 'putting one foot in front of the other'), and a wide base (indicative of sensory or cerebellar disease).

Step 3: mental status examination. The neurological examination must include evaluation of mental status and level of consciousness. The former is essential in routine care of the elderly. Otherwise, a patient with early dementia may fool the examiner by maintaining a competent 'social demeanor' and concealing deficits with approximate answers, bantering or changes of topic. There are several useful tools for this purpose.

Mini mental state examination (MMSE). For all but the most severely impaired, the cognitive mental state can be usefully assessed using a standardized inventory of cognitive capacities such as the MMSE. The MMSE is brief and simple enough for use in routine office practice with older patients, yet is sufficiently comprehensive that, when combined with other clinical measures, it provides a valuable index of the severity and staging of dementia (Table 5.1).

The MMSE probes five cognitive 'domains'. The first section covers orientation, memory, attention and concentration. Memory is tested by noting the number of trials required to learn three object names then testing recall later. Attention and concentration are tested by the serial subtraction of 7s from 100, or by spelling the word 'world' backwards. The next questions test for loss of ability to:

- repeat a simple spoken phrase (language fluency)
- name common objects (nominal aphasia)
- follow a three-stage verbal command (receptive aphasia, apraxia)
- comprehend and follow a one-stage written command (alexia)
- write a sentence spontaneously (aphasia, apraxia).

The test is completed by asking the patient to copy a simple figure of two intersecting pentagons (constructional apraxia). The maximum score is 30 points. A score of less than 24 is broadly indicative of cognitive impairment. However, this threshold is not universal – individuals of lower original mental ability are likely to achieve lower scores, whereas those with superior intellect will typically do better. For example, a score of 27 or less in a university graduate would probably suggest cognitive impairment.

National Adult Reading Test (NART). This simple test may be useful for estimation of the premorbid mental ability, and hence the differentiation of dementia (which implies decline) from longstanding cognitive deficit. The patient is asked to read aloud a standard list of words with irregular spellings. For example, someone who had not encountered the word 'syncope' might be unaware of the conventional emphasis placed on the last letter. The test comprises 50 such words of

TABLE 5.1

Mini mental state examination (MMSE) questions

1. Orientation

(Score 1 for correct, 0 for incorrect)

What is the year we are in?

What season is it?

What is today's date?

What day of the week is it today?

What month are we in?

What county are we in?

What country (or state) are we in?

What town are we in?

Can you tell me the name of this place?

What floor of the building are we on?

2. Registration

Ask the patient if you may test their memory. Then say the names of three unrelated objects, clearly and slowly, about 1 second for each, 'lemon, key, ball'. After the patient has said all three, ask them to repeat the objects. The first repetition determines the score (0–3) but keep saying them until the patient can repeat all three, up to five trials. If the patient does not eventually learn all three, recall cannot be meaningfully tested. (Score 0–3)

3. Attention and calculation

Ask the patient to begin with 100 and subtract 7, and then to keep subtracting 7s. Stop after five subtractions (93,86,79,72,65). Score the number of answers that represented the prior answer minus 7. Ask the patient to spell the word 'world' backwards. The score is the number of letters in correct order (e.g. dlrow = 5, dlorw = 3). Record the higher score of the two tasks. (Score 0–5)

4. Recall

Ask the patient if they can recall the three words you previously asked them to remember. (Score 0–3)

CONTINUED

TABLE 5.1 (CONTINUED)

5. Naming

(a) Show the patient a wristwatch and ask them what it is.

(b) Repeat for a pencil.

(Score 0–2)

6. Repetition

Ask the patient to repeat this phrase after you word-for-word: 'No ifs, ands or buts'. Allow only one trial. (Score 0–1)

7. Three-stage command

Have the patient follow this command: 'Take a paper in your (non-dominant) hand, fold it in half using both hands and put it on the floor'. Score one point for each part correctly executed. (Score 0–3)

8. Reading

On a blank piece of paper print the sentence 'Close your eyes' in letters large enough for the patient to see clearly. Ask the patient to read it and do what it says. Score 1 point only if they actually close their eyes. (Score 0–1)

9. Writing

Give the patient a blank piece of paper and ask them to write a sentence for you. Do not dictate a sentence, it is to be written spontaneously. It must contain a subject and a verb and be sensible. Correct grammar and punctuation are not necessary. (Score 0–1)

10. Copying

On a clean piece of paper, draw intersecting pentagons, and ask the patient to copy it. All ten angles must be present, and two angles must intersect to score 1 point. Ignore tremor and rotation. (Score 0–1)

Maximum score: 30

Source: *J Psychiatr Res* 1975;12:189–98

decreasing familiarity. It can be administered quickly and correlates well with original intelligence quotient.

Briefer mental tests for non-specialist use. The MMSE can be shortened for use in primary care with little loss of specificity. Items retained in the short version include:

- orientation to day of the week
- spell the word 'world' backwards
- recall three words after a delay of 1 minute with distraction
- the request to write a proper sentence.

Another reliable indicator of dementia is a carer's account of deterioration in four activities of daily living, including:

- managing medication
- using the telephone
- coping with a budget
- using transport.

These eight items can be easily incorporated into a routine domiciliary consultation, together with the clock-drawing test (Figure 5.1), which also has good sensitivity and specificity for dementia. It is strongly recommended that family physicians use and record these formal cognitive test procedures as a minimum in their evaluation of dementia, particularly when evaluating and monitoring the effects of pharmacological treatments for dementia. On a cautionary note, however, scores from these tests should not be preferred to a clear statement of the likely diagnosis and prognosis. Great care must be exercised when a patient scores well on a dementia screening test but the history is strongly suggestive of dementia. Some atypical forms of Alzheimer's disease and several frontal type dementias can present with relatively few cognitive signs and/or preserved verbal memory; in these instances a 'normal' screening score does not imply that the patient does not have dementia.

Assessment of delirium or altered consciousness. This is another important aspect of examining mental status. The diagnosis of a cognitive disorder should always include consideration of delirium (see pages 32–4). Informal quantitative assessment of attention and concentration may be useful. Another valuable test is to ask the patient, if cooperative, to extend both arms, then fully dorsiflex the hands and hold this awkward posture. The clinician may demonstrate, or assist the patient to achieve the desired posture, but then let go. Delirious

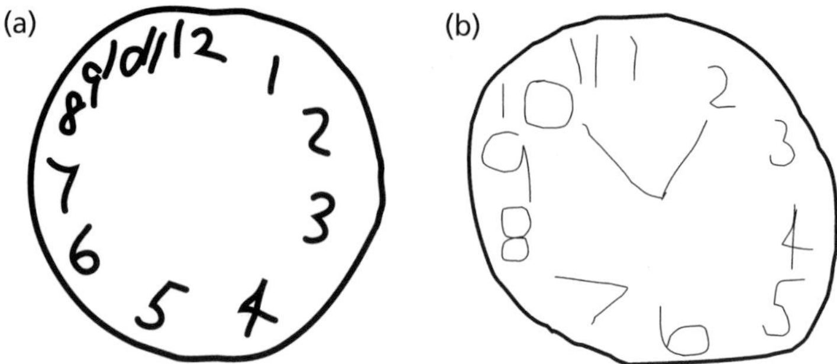

Figure 5.1 The clock-drawing test. (a) Exaggerated spacing of low numbers leads to crowding of high numbers. (b) The patient was instructed to 'Draw a clock face and set the hands to ten past eleven'. Number 12 is missing.

patients (not only those with hepatic encephalopathy) often exhibit asterixis – irregular myoclonic jerking movements of the entire hand or selected digits.

Step 4: assessment of disordered emotion and behavior. There is good evidence that behavioral and emotional concomitants of dementia are as important as cognitive state in predicting burden of care, need for residential placement, etc. Several instruments have therefore been introduced to enable comprehensive and uniform assessment of behavioral symptoms in dementia.

The Neuropsychiatric Inventory (NPI) introduced by Cummings and colleagues is the best known of these. It is a structured interview for administration to a carer or other party who is familiar with the patient's behavioral repertoire. Its most widely used version has ten sections covering: hallucinations, delusions, agitation/anxiety, depressed mood, apathy, irritability or aggressive behaviors, stereotyped or repetitive purposeless behaviors, resistiveness to care, and socially inappropriate behaviors. Each section includes a 'probe' question to be asked verbatim. Positive responses are followed up with specific questions intended to elaborate specific behaviors, and then further questions to establish the frequency and severity of these behavioral difficulties. A final panel of questions inquires about changes in sleep, appetite, energy level, and expressed sexual interests. This instrument is especially useful for monitoring the effect of behavioral or pharmacological interventions.

Step 5: assessment of functional capacity. Functional capacity and cognitive abilities do not always go hand in hand. An important part of the evaluation for dementia is therefore an assessment of the patient's abilities in ordinary activities of daily living. Apart from the simple questions described above, several measures are available to facilitate this assessment. These include the Short Blessed test of activities of daily living and the dementia symptom rating scale (DSRS). Because there may occasionally be an unusual degree of dissociation between cognitive abilities and functional state, these tests are useful metrics for the latter.

Step 6: diagnostic imaging. Until recently, consensus groups had not recommended routine structural imaging using CT or magnetic resonance imaging (MRI) in the early investigation of dementia. Now, however, these procedures have been recommended, if available, as an aid to differential diagnosis and management decisions. CT is generally sufficient to exclude intracerebral pathology (tumor, hematoma, hydrocephalus), and the newer higher resolution scanners permit a crude assessment of deep cortical and white-matter changes in tissue composition ('leukoaraiosis') that may reflect chronic vascular or perfusion deficits. MRI provides greater structural information, including estimates of hippocampal atrophy, frontotemporal lobar degeneration and, in particular, a more precise assessment of the location and extent of vascular lesions. Even in the absence of dementia, white-matter lesions may be associated with cognitive deficits, including slowed processing, immediate and delayed memory and overall impairment of planning and mental function. Although the yield from these imaging techniques in the discovery of treatable conditions is low (certainly less than 10% and possibly less than 1%), they do often reveal useful information about the cause and likely course of the patient's cognitive deficit. Unless extensive, however, atrophy alone is of uncertain value in the diagnosis of dementia (see Figure 2.1, page 21).

Step 7: other optional or specialized measures. In the USA, positron emission tomography (PET) with the metabolic marker fluorodexyglucose is now used for differential diagnosis of early or ambiguous instances of cognitive disorder. There is a characteristic alteration in ratio of metabolic activity in frontal versus temporoparietal regions that can strongly suggest Alzheimer's disease. At present, PET imaging is available only in a few specialized centers. Single photon emission computed tomography (SPECT) may be considered for similar identification of regional metabolic disturbance (e.g. in differentiating Alzheimer's disease from frontal lobe dementia), but this method is less precise and should not be the sole imaging investigation for dementia.

The electroencephalogram (EEG) may be useful in particular circumstances but is not needed for evaluation of most typical cases of dementia. The EEG can be diagnostic in Creutzfeldt–Jakob disease (CJD), showing periodic sharp complexes, but these are not always present and may disappear as the dementia progresses. Novel research

Key points – clinical examination and investigations

- Initial assessment must include a careful clinical history and investigations to detect causes of reversible ('treatable') dementia.
- All initial assessments should record an estimate of dementia severity and be based on a method for which age- and education-standardized normal ('non-demented') values are available.
- In community-based clinical practice, simple formal tests of cognitive function and activities of daily living should be performed and recorded. In specialist practice, standardized behavioral and emotional ratings should be used routinely.
- SPECT and other metabolic imaging may help distinguish between Alzheimer's disease and predominantly vascular dementia. The place of brain structural imaging techniques in the routine assessment of dementia is uncertain.

methods of EEG analysis are also being investigated as diagnostic tools in dementia. These rely on the fact that the electrical activity of the brain is highly synchronized in support of the coordination necessary between specialized brain areas to accomplish cognitive tasks. EEG measures are non-invasive and highly quantifiable. EEG data may prove most useful when combined with structural imaging.

There are no well-established indications for molecular genetic studies (e.g. apolipoprotein E genotype; see Chapter 9) in current routine clinical practice. Where an impressive family history of dementia is reported, referral to specialist genetic advisory services may be made.

Key references

Jacoby R, Oppenheimer C, Dening T, Thomas A, eds. *Oxford Textbook of Old Age Psychiatry*, 4th edn. Oxford: Oxford University Press, 2008.

Heinik J, Reider-Groswasser II, Solomesh I et al. Clock drawing test: correlation with linear measurements of CT studies in demented patients. *Int J Geriatr Psychiatry* 2000; 15:1130–7.

Knopman DS, DeKosky ST, Cummings JL et al. Practice parameter: Diagnosis of dementia (an evidence-based review). Report of the Quality Standards Subcommittee of the American Academy of Neurology. *Neurology* 2001;56: 1143–53.

Konno S, Meyer JS, Terayama Y et al. Classification, diagnosis and treatment of vascular dementia. *Drugs Aging* 1997;11:361–73.

Lund and Manchester Groups. Clinical and neuropathological criteria for frontotemporal dementia. *J Neurol Neurosurg Psychiatry* 1994;57:416–18.

McKeith IG, Gakasji D, Kosaka K et al. Consensus guidelines for the clinical and pathologic diagnosis of dementia with Lewy bodies (DLB): report of the consortium on DLB international workshop. *Neurology* 1996;47:1113–24.

McKhann G, Drachman D, Folstein M et al. Clinical diagnosis of Alzheimer's disease: report of the NINCDS-ADRDA Work Group under the auspices of Department of Health and Human Services Task Force on Alzheimer's Disease. *Neurology* 1984;34:939–44.

Nathan J, Wilkinson D, Stammers S, Low JL. The role of tests of frontal executive function in the detection of mild dementia. *Int J Geriatr Psychiatry* 2001;16:18–26.

Pasquier F. Early diagnosis of dementia: neuropsychology. *J Neurol* 1999;246:6–15.

Rabins PV, Lyketsos CG, Steele CD. *Practical Dementia Care*, 2nd edn. New York: Oxford University Press, 2006.

Roman GC, Tatemichi TK, Erkiunjuntti T et al. Vascular dementia: diagnostic criteria for research studies. Report of the NINDS-AIREN International Workshop. *Neurology* 1993;43: 250–60.

Walstra GJM, Teunisse S, vanGool WA et al. Reversible dementia in elderly patients referred to a memory clinic. *J Neurol* 1997; 244:17–22.

6 Principles of care and treatment

Delivering the dementia diagnosis

Family physicians are often the first point of contact with health services for a patient with dementia. Most physicians can exclude any physical disease that accounts for the presentation, and can identify reversible causes of dementia when present. At this point, the health professional must consider how best to disclose the initial diagnosis.

The eminent Scottish geriatrician Sir Ferguson Anderson was fond of saying, "The greatest gift that a physician can give his patient is a diagnosis – provided, of course, that it is the correct diagnosis." Early in the course of dementia care it is therefore useful to establish with caregivers and patients the most probable causes for the presentation. Many patients are aware of the differential diagnostic possibilities for dementia, and they may sometimes ask awkward questions. Sir Ferguson once suggested that answers should be "an edited version of the truth", but members of the clinical team must consider how much 'editing' is in the patient's best interest. It is fairly common to give a patient with early dementia good advice to help plan the next few years, and perhaps to influence treatment. Caregivers should be made fully aware of likely diagnoses and their implications for future personal safety and independence.

The diagnostic review interview. The first step in this process is to set a time with the patient when the results of the assessment can be discussed and decisions can be made as to what might happen thereafter. There the examining physician will either confirm the dementia diagnosis or, if this is still uncertain, he/she will describe the extra information that is needed for a more secure diagnosis, having first determined how much of that information should be available to the patient and to the caregiver. The physician can decide how much information to disclose by understanding:

- the principal fears of both patient and caregiver
- what the patient knows about dementia, its causes and courses

- the nature of any family history of dementia (about which the patient may have already drawn conclusions)
- the likely resilience of the patient when presented with a dementia diagnosis.

Although rare, extreme emotional reactions to a dementia diagnosis should be anticipated in vulnerable individuals, and thought should be given to the acute management of these patients in the clinic. Three key aspects of the decision to disclose the dementia diagnosis are:

- what does the patient already know?
- what are the benefits of the patient knowing more?
- what are the hazards of disclosure?

The diagnostic review interview brings together all that the physician and caregiver know about the patient, assesses the impact of the diagnosis on the patient and stresses that the diagnosis is only a first step. It is not essential to share the results of specific investigations (e.g. cortical atrophy detected on brain imaging) to convince the patient that dementia is present; it is simpler to agree and to help reconcile the patient with the need for further investigations and possible treatment. Some patients will be reassured by the care taken to understand fully the nature of their difficulties. Patients with early dementia will often retain the ability to report failings of memory and may be relieved to discover that the problems they have been experiencing are not simply 'old age' and are probably caused by an underlying brain illness. These patients are likely to acknowledge the need for investigation and, eventually, the importance of diagnosis.

Occasionally, however, the discussion of the diagnosis is more complicated: patients and/or caregivers may deny problems possibly attributable to dementia, making light of issues that clearly indicate a serious underlying problem. In these circumstances, time should be set aside to understand the causes of their denial and to seek ways that ensure appropriate investigations take place and results are discussed with the patient. It is important to be aware that caregivers can be inconsistent in their views about disclosure of a dementia diagnosis; for example, they may argue that a patient should not be told even though they are often adamant that if they were the patient they would wish to be fully informed.

As a general rule, because our understanding of dementing illnesses remains imprecise and the clinical diagnosis is typically provisional, it is often reassuring (and truthful) to say that a more certain diagnosis will only be possible after an interval (e.g. 6 months).

The clinical assistant's role. If possible, a diagnostic review should be conducted in the presence of a clinical assistant, usually a clinic nurse. After the patient has received the discouraging news, the assistant may offer to meet with the patient and caregiver to discuss the diagnosis, to assess educational needs about dementia and dementia services, and to initiate a process of caring that acknowledges the need for practical help and how to get it. Patients may need help in responding to emotional reactions to the diagnosis. Family members often express concerns about managing money, legal issues and social security (welfare) benefits, and have worries about physical safety and general health; they will want to know how to plan for the future. Otherwise, such matters are easily overlooked in a busy clinic. In some centers, specific dementia management protocols include these issues as critical aspects of dementia care, often restated in educational material given to the patient and caregiver at the time of diagnosis (Table 6.1). This type of information should be available in all clinics. The Internet, voluntary organizations and health service agencies are excellent sources of educational material (see Useful addresses, page 113).

Hazards of disclosure. Risk of self-harm and suicide are increased in individuals recently diagnosed with dementia. Risk factors for suicide in dementia patients include depressed mood, retained insight, young age at presentation and, later in dementia, failure to respond to anti-dementia drugs. The examining physician should be as aware as possible of these risks, and should routinely record an examination of the patient's mental state that includes questioning about depressed mood, feelings of hopelessness, despair or any dwelling on the idea that suicide might be 'the only way out'. Some of these issues are difficult to assess and in these circumstances a caregiver can provide valuable insights into the patient's views about his/her symptoms and, potentially, known wishes if affected by dementia. It is helpful to record

TABLE 6.1

Checklist of educational materials to support dementia patients and their caregivers

- Knowledge about dementia
  - What is dementia?
  - How often does dementia progress?
  - What treatments are available?
  - Does treatment work?
- Emotions and dementia
  - Where are the words to express how you feel when dementia strikes?
  - The roles of caregiver, family and friends
  - Sharing care and knowing when you need help
- Money matters
  - Financial planning
  - Social security (welfare) benefits
  - Assets and protection of the dementia patient
  - How to get help to fill in forms
- Legal powers
  - Adults with incapacity legislation
  - Role of the court (guardianship and other legal interventions)
  - Power of attorney
  - Making a will
  - Wishes about future medical treatment ('advance directives' and 'living wills')
- Practical aspects of caring
  - Physical health
  - Mental activity
  - Spiritual well-being
- Activities of daily living
  - Personal hygiene
  - Dressing
  - Continence
  - Nutritional status
- Unwanted behaviors
  - Wandering
  - Shouting
  - Aggression
  - Sexual interest and intimacy
- Safety
  - Hazards at home
  - Driving
  - Alcohol and drugs

these fears about diagnosis and to try, in cooperation with the caregiver, to anticipate the patient's likely reaction to a dementia diagnosis.

Sometimes the diagnosis must be broached with great care – potentially over several meetings – with inclusion of assurances of confidentiality and future support. When faced with possible denial of a dementia diagnosis, it is useful to consider whether the patient's views about dementia might influence their reaction to this outcome. In anticipation of this it is good practice to ensure, from the time of presentation, that the patient and caregiver have access to good quality information about the causes of the patient's symptoms, what investigations are most useful and a guide to treatment decisions (see Table 6.1).

Ongoing assessment

In addition to formal diagnostic assessment, good clinical practice includes the assessment of continuing abilities to perform domestic chores and to drive a car, as well as an estimation of likely risk of self-injury because of failing cognitive ability. Figure 6.1 shows the types of

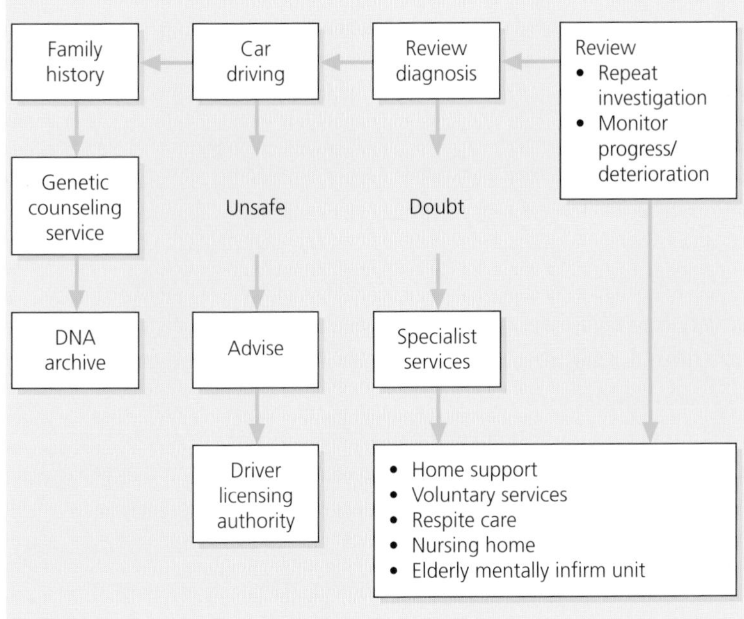

Figure 6.1 Decisions made by a dementia care team.

decision made by a dementia care team. Usually, a patient and caregiver accept advice when car driving has become unsafe. The message may be reinforced by pointing out the possibility not only of self-injury but also of harm to others. The potential threat of legal liability and insurance issues may further accentuate the point.

Diagnostic follow-up. As discussed above, it is good practice to include in the management plan a date for formal diagnostic follow-up. This is often carried out 6 months after presentation but it may be up to a year later. This follow-up visit can be helpful for caregivers, particularly if no active treatment plan was initiated when diagnostic assessment was first completed. The rate of change or decline in cognition and function becomes a paramount issue in longitudinal care, and the follow-up visit provides an opportunity to assess this using the mini mental state examination (MMSE), the cornerstone for monitoring cognitive symptoms (see pages 52–4), or similar measures.

The patient's recollection of medical recommendations may also have faded with time, even when initially well understood, so this is an opportunity to reiterate the treatment plan.

Occasionally the course of an apparent dementia will be atypical and suggest other diagnoses. This is particularly important when initial presentation was complicated by use of sedative drugs, a confusional state or exacerbation of a systemic illness. Medical review also provides an opportunity to evaluate the quality of care received. Sometimes a doctor or nurse is the only independent person able to do this on behalf of the patient. Furthermore, it is occasionally necessary to draw attention to exploitation or even physical abuse of a patient with dementia; diagnostic follow-up provides a good opportunity to make relevant observations.

Decisions about brain imaging, disclosure of diagnosis, unsafe car driving, genetic counseling, the management of behavioral complications of dementia, and the introduction of anti-dementia drugs such as galantamine, rivastigmine and donepezil, are either deferred to secondary care or form part of a sequence of decisions offered by the general or geriatric physician and care team (see Figure 6.1). Likewise, decisions must be made about procedures to monitor care and response to drugs.

Pain and dementia

Pain is common in old age, and is therefore also a problem for patients with dementia. More than 60% of nursing-home residents make frequent complaints of pain. Not surprisingly, chronic or recurrent pain is an important cause of sleeplessness and agitation. In dementia, impairments of memory, reasoning and (especially) language often impair the patient's capacity to report pain, and observational measures are required to assess pain. A key initial step is therefore to evaluate the needs of clinical staff (including nurses' aides) for training in pain recognition and care. Many nursing-home residents, including those whose use of language is impaired, *can* provide consistent and reliable self-reported pain data when they receive sufficient time and assistance, relying on any of several pain assessment instruments.

A number of score sheets are easily used and trusted in dementia care. Table 6.2 shows the Abbey pain scale, but other equally useful scales are available. In dementia, as elsewhere, standard step therapy is the basis of pain management (see Chapter 7). A patient with dementia who is in severe pain – who may be noisy and frightened as a result – challenges the skills of the clinical team and it is not unreasonable to adopt an empirical approach to analgesia. The benefits of treatment should be demonstrated by improvement in pain scores on a standardized instrument (see Table 6.2) that includes recording changes in physical, psychosocial and cognitive functions. Optimum pain management can improve these functional domains and the quality of life of a nursing-home resident.

Adequate nutrition

Assessment of nutritional status is a key component of the examination of health in the elderly. Poor nutrition and lifestyle changes may increase the risk of loss of tissue function, and of diseases such as atherosclerosis and osteoporosis. Although total energy requirements are lower in the elderly (1800–2100 kcal/day in men; 400 kcal fewer in women), there is widespread evidence that old people typically eat 10% less than this. Food frequency estimates based on usual dietary habits are notoriously unreliable in cognitively impaired subjects. There is also good evidence that old people receiving community care services are undernourished,

TABLE 6.2

The Abbey pain scale for measurement of pain in people with dementia who cannot verbalize; the scale should be completed while the patient is observed

Time since last pain relief administered: .... (hours)					
Category	Signs (score)	Absent (0)	Mild (1)	Moderate (2)	Severe (3)
Vocalization	Whimpering, groaning, crying				
Facial expression	Looking tense or frightened, frowning, grimacing				
Change in body language	Fidgeting, rocking, guarding part of the body, withdrawn				
Behavioral change	Increased confusion, refusing to eat, alteration in usual patterns				
Physiological change	Temperature, pulse or blood pressure outside normal limits, perspiring, flushing, pallor				
Physical changes	Skin tears, pressure areas, arthritis, contractures, previous injuries				
Total score	*Add all scores from above*				
Pain severity		0–2 (No pain)	3–7 (Mild)	8–13 (Moderate)	14+ (Severe)
Type of pain	Chronic	Acute		Acute on chronic	

Adapted from Abbey J et al. 2004.

and the same is often true of old people in residential care. Low bodyweight (detected as body mass index, BMI, below 20 kg/m^2) and progressive weight loss are readily detected. Careful inquiry sometimes reveals low intake of energy (in terms of total calories), protein and antioxidant vitamins, vitamin B_{12} and folate. Patients with dementia are at high risk of malnutrition, both at home and in residential care.

When patients are poorly nourished, steps should be taken to improve diet and to measure response to that intervention. Recommended daily dietary allowances for old people can be used to optimize nutrition. This is particularly important when poor diet and poverty coexist. When total food consumption is low, intake of essential vitamins can be quickly marginalized in old people. The use of vitamin and fish-oil supplements is commonplace among health-conscious old people. There is some preliminary evidence (mostly from prospective observational studies) that dietary supplements promote retention of cognitive function in late life, and one randomized controlled trial suggests that supplementation with supraphysiological doses of α-tocopherol (vitamin E) will delay time to obligatory residential care in patients with late-onset Alzheimer's disease.

Epidemiological studies confirm the importance of a good balanced diet to the maintenance of health in old age. The discovery that homocysteine is a risk factor for dementia (see page 91) lends weight to the nutritional argument that too little attention is paid to the promotion of adequate intake of folate and vitamin B_{12}. The theoretical dangers of neuronal damage resulting from the unopposed effects of folate are too slight to cause concerns about the addition of folate to cereals and other foodstuffs. There is also some evidence from longitudinal observational studies that a diet rich in fish oils (omega-3 fatty acids) with adequate antioxidants has brain-protective benefits.

There are also data to suggest a lower incidence of dementia where the consumption of fish oils forms a significant part of the diet compared with vegetable oils (omega-6 fatty acids).

Behavioral problems

The management of behavioral problems in dementia is based on sound and consistent nursing and prescribing practice. Whenever possible, those involved in the care of people with dementia should be fully aware of local procedures. In nursing homes and dementia care units, these procedures should be written down and reviewed regularly. When an unwanted behavior is detected, caregivers should be encouraged to look for 'triggers' in the patient's circumstances that may be linked to onset or offset; these may include physiological sensations like the need to urinate. Simple reassurance often helps allay the fears of desertion or harm prompted by anxiety or uncertainty. Unfortunately for many caregivers, such reassurance may lead to intense feelings of dependency on the part of the dementia patient, who may seek the near-continuous comforting presence of the caregiver. In such circumstances, skilled support may be necessary to afford the caregiver some respite. Table 6.3 shows non-drug interventions for behavioral problems in dementia.

Medication should be considered only after psychological and educational strategies have failed, and the introduction of drugs must be balanced against their possible adverse effects. For sedative drugs, these effects include an apparent worsening of dementia, falls, cumulative toxicity, tolerance and withdrawal phenomena, and extrapyramidal side effects. The last are particularly troubling for dementia patients because their distress can sometimes be ignored when language is impaired and effects like akathisia or drooling are wrongly attributed to dementia rather than the medication.

When drugs are used, attention should be paid to the patient's understanding and consent to treatment, drug choice, dosage and duration. Subterfuge, coercion or physical restraint should not be used to administer a drug unless approved by a properly constituted authority that is legally permitted to grant such approval. It is better to avoid sedative drugs, particularly benzodiazepines, whenever possible. If there is no alternative, these drugs should be used at the lowest effective

TABLE 6.3

Non-drug interventions for behavioral problems in dementia

- Reality orientation
  Accurate information about person and surroundings
- Behavioral analysis
  Detailed analysis of behavior, content and triggers
- Occupational activities
  Positive stimulation, e.g. music therapy
- Environmental modifications
  Changes in care routines, orientation cues
- Sensory stimulation
  Touch/massage, aromatherapy, bright light
- Education
  Carer-focused, social support measures

dose and withdrawn within 1 month. Generally, older dementia patients are more sensitive to the adverse effects of drugs used to control behavioral symptoms or signs. It is good practice to start at the lowest dose and increase gradually at intervals of at least five times the half-life of the selected drug. Whenever possible, drug prescribing guidelines should be agreed in residential facilities. A useful rule is 'start low, go slow'. Medical review of prescribing should include steps to detect inadvertent or deliberate administration to the patient of drugs intended for another (perhaps a caregiver or fellow resident).

Progression and age of onset

The natural history of dementing illnesses will conform approximately to the prognosis linked to each specific dementia diagnosis. Later age at onset is generally associated with a slower progression; younger adults with dementia are more likely to progress quickly. Where vascular brain pathologies are important, progress is often slow in between abrupt periods of worsening and increased confusion that reflect new vascular insults.

Caregivers will often ask about future care and seek advice about residential care with a view to ensuring the dementia patient's quality of life is preserved. Answers to these and related questions require knowledge of local care facilities and an appreciation of the wishes of the patient. Usually it is reasonable to presume that the rate of deterioration will remain relatively constant, such that ratings of dementia severity will change by roughly equal steps over successive 6-month intervals. This assumption relates to a clinical 'rule of thumb' that:

- the MMSE score will decline, on average, by 3 points every year
- MMSE scores above 18 are often compatible with independent living
- MMSE scores below 13 usually indicate a need for careful daily supervision.

When reliable change scores like these are recorded they form a basis of useful discussions with caregivers about rates of change and the impact (if any) of treatment effects.

Managing treatment expectations

Physicians are frequently asked questions about cognitive enhancement treatments. If dementia patients score more than 12 points on the MMSE, a therapeutic trial of a cholinesterase inhibitor should be discussed (see Chapter 7). However, expectations of treatment benefits should not be exaggerated, and it is important to emphasize how difficult it can be to predict an individual's response. It is worth noting, nonetheless, that a few patients do experience a dramatic response to these drugs. The physician should also emphasize that the treatment is symptomatic and will probably not modify the underlying brain disease. Figure 6.2 shows that when symptomatic treatment is withdrawn the pattern of progress returns to the point of decline predicted had treatment not been introduced. In contrast, if a disease-modifying anti-dementia drug were to be withdrawn the decline in dementia would run in parallel with the natural history of the illness, any advantage of the drug remaining as a lag in progress linked in time to duration of exposure to the drug. This latter scenario remains hypothetical as currently available anti-dementia drugs provide symptomatic improvement only and do not address the underlying pathology of the illness.

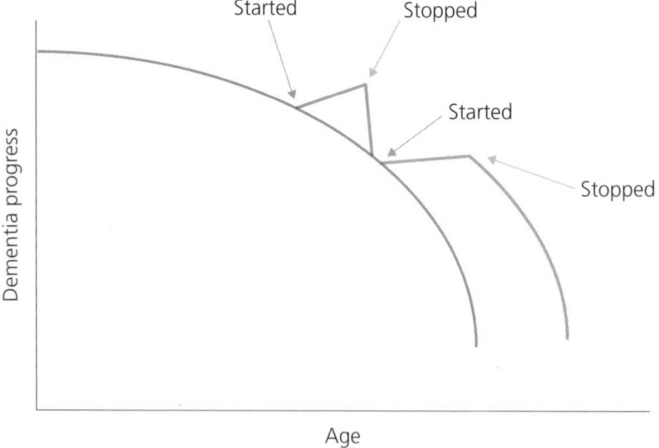

Figure 6.2 The curved line shows the natural progression of untreated dementia with age. When symptomatic treatment (————) is started there is an improvement but when it is withdrawn the pattern of progress returns to the same point of decline had treatment not been introduced. In contrast, if a disease-modifying anti-dementia drug (————) were to be withdrawn the decline in dementia would run in parallel with the natural history of the illness.

Some national guidelines encourage the withdrawal of anticholinesterase drugs when patients deteriorate so much that they score less than 12 on the MMSE. Naturalistic studies support the clinical view that – despite the emphasis placed by those who promulgate these guidelines – the effects of anticholinesterase withdrawal may considerably disadvantage the individual patient. Flying in the face of the confidence expressed in national guidelines, some clinicians stress the importance of considering each patient carefully and judging the impact of drug withdrawal on the patient's quality of life, the caregiver's burden and, sometimes, the risks of increased mortality. Most agree there is a need for new research on cholinesterase inhibitors in the severe stage of dementia and on changing and withdrawing medication safely in these patients. More neurobiological research is needed to determine the long-term changes on transmitter sensitivities as a result of taking cholinesterase inhibitors.

Clinical surveillance in residential care

Unfortunately, it is not uncommon for dementia patients to enter long-term residential care and thereafter to receive few visitors who might have known the patient before dementia onset. A visiting physician is usually called to attend when physical health deteriorates or behavior becomes unmanageable. Because trained labor constitutes a major cost in residential care, some care homes employ the least number of trained caregivers and rely on workers who may receive little support or training, remaining on hand only for short periods. Some caution is required by the visiting physician in residential care. Critical areas that require clinical vigilance are:

- nutritional status
- elder abuse
- drowsiness and despondency.

Nutritional status. Feeding practices should be noted. Staff need to be trained to help feed high-dependency patients; typically, patients require 20 minutes individual attention at each meal with care being taken to ensure that warm food is palatable. The monthly weights of all patients should be recorded.

Elder abuse is not confined to residential care. The abuser is usually someone known to the patient. When health workers become involved, it is more usual for one worker to 'target' the victimized patient rather

Key points – principles of care and treatment

- When considering disclosure of the dementia diagnosis, the physician should take into account what the patient already knows, the benefits of the patient knowing more and the hazards associated with disclosure.
- If possible, a diagnostic review interview should be conducted in the presence of a clinical assistant, usually a clinic nurse, who will be able to acknowledge and assist with the need for practical help and how to get it once the diagnosis has been made; care is best provided by a dementia team with a range of skills to investigate, treat and support patients and caregivers.
- In dementia, impaired memory, reasoning and (especially) language often prevent the patient reporting pain, so observational measures are required to assess pain; optimum pain management can improve the physical, psychosocial, cognitive functions and overall quality of life of elderly dementia patients.
- Nutritional status is a key part of assessment; signs and symptoms of dementia may improve when nutrition is optimized.
- Drug treatments of behavioral symptoms should only be used after non-drug interventions have failed. When used, medication should be initiated at a low dose, with the dose increased slowly if necessary ('start low, go slow').
- For those with mild-to-moderate dementia in whom the presence of Alzheimer-type pathology seems likely, treatment with an acetylcholinesterase inhibitor should be considered, irrespective of age.
- Expectations of treatment benefits should not be exaggerated. The physician should emphasize that the treatment is symptomatic and will probably not modify the underlying brain disease.

than the care home to have an institutionalized but unwritten policy of abuse. Physical abuse is the easiest to detect, usually from tell-tale bruising of areas commonly used for restraint. Signs of neglect and psychological, financial and sexual abuse are much more difficult to detect on occasional visits but should be looked for as part of the routine inspection of care homes by those responsible for their accreditation.

Drowsiness and despondency are often attributable to progressive dementia but can be linked to sedative use. It is unsafe to assume that drug administration in residential care is conducted and supervised to a standard expected in hospital inpatient care. Compounding drug administration is the problem of inadvertent (and sometimes covert) administration of drugs to a patient other than the person for whom the medication is intended.

Key references

Abbey J, Piller N, De Bellis A et al. The Abbey pain scale: a 1-minute numerical indicator for people with end-stage dementia *Int J Palliat Nurs* 2004;10:6–13.

Haw C, Harwood D, Hawton K. Dementia and suicidal behavior: a review of the literature. *Int Psychogeriatr* 2009;21:440–53.

Jacoby R, Oppenheimer C, Dening T, Thomas A, eds. *Oxford Textbook of Old Age Psychiatry*, 4th edn. Oxford: Oxford University Press, 2008.

Pinner G, Bouman W-P; What should we tell people about dementia? *Adv Psychiatr Treat* 2003;9:335–41.

Rabins PV, Lyketsos CG, Steele CD. *Practical Dementia Care*, 2nd edn. New York: Oxford University Press, 2006.

7 Pharmacological treatment

Acetylcholinesterase inhibitors

The cholinergic system is important in learning and memory. The idea that the functions of cholinergic neurons are essential to learning and memory is supported by studies of surgical lesions of cholinergic fibers in animals, pharmacological studies of anticholinergic agents, and neurochemical studies in aging and Alzheimer's disease. Between 1972 and 1980, such studies laid the basis for almost two decades of therapeutic research on the cholinergic system in Alzheimer's disease. At first, it appeared that reduced cholinergic function was specific for Alzheimer's disease and was not found in other types of dementia. However, in cross-diagnostic studies with adequate control samples, most postmortem studies of brain tissues found that levels of enzymes associated with the synthesis (choline acetyl transferase, ChAT) and degradation (acetylcholinesterase, AChE) of acetylcholine were reduced not only in Alzheimer's disease but also, to a lesser extent, in aging in the absence of dementia, alcoholic dementia, dementia associated with Parkinson's disease and in some instances of vascular dementia. Thus, the conclusion that the cholinergic deficit was specific to Alzheimer's disease was abandoned.

Over the past 30 years, many attempts have been made to enhance cholinergic function in Alzheimer's disease. Compounds that contained precursors of acetylcholine or mimicked its actions in the brain were tested, but none proved successful. By contrast, AChE inhibitors provide a sound foundation to the pharmacological management of dementia and are now the first line of drug treatment for Alzheimer's disease. Three drugs are currently available in most countries: donepezil, galantamine and rivastigmine. Their pharmacological profiles are broadly similar, but there are some important differences in pharmocokinetic properties and information on safety and benefits in routine clinical practice.

The case was convincingly made by manufacturers, and accepted by licensing authorities, that this group of drugs is of potential benefit to a substantial proportion of individuals with mild-to-moderate Alzheimer's disease. The economic case for the drugs was not based simply on change in cognition; it was closely linked to the problem of disability in old people. Cognitive function is a major determinant of disability in old age – so much so that about 40% of disabled people aged 65 years and over and about 50% of people in institutional care have cognitive impairment; this impairment is now the main reason for such care. Dementia also contributes to hospitalization and disability in other ways. For example, a reduction in dementia prevalence of 1–2% would probably reduce the number of hip fractures in the UK by 20 000 per year.

Rates for the institutionalization of patients with dementia vary widely between localities; in general, dementia patients are about four times more likely to move into institutional care than age-matched people with intact cognition. About 30% of patients who attend a memory clinic typically move into residential care within a year of first attending the clinic. These moves are explained by progressive functional decline that can be readily quantitated by activities of daily living (ADL) scores.

The AChE inhibitors can reduce disability and institutionalization rates. One early study of patients receiving tacrine (no longer widely used) showed that doses above 80 mg/day reduced the likelihood of admission to a nursing home compared with lower doses or those who had stopped taking the drug. Analysis of the complex tasks component of an ADL measure collected during a double-blind randomized controlled trial of donepezil showed that active treatment groups improved when compared with placebo, with statistical significance for the 10 mg/day dose of donepezil. Subjects who tolerated a daily dose of 6 mg or more of rivastigmine had unchanged personal ADL scores over 6 months, while those receiving either less than 6 mg or placebo experienced significant decline.

Rivastigmine doses of at least 6 mg daily reduce institutionalization by 8–14% per year. This percentage compares favorably with an absolute reduction of 1.5% as an acceptable benefit of stroke unit care. At the time of writing, there have been 13 randomized placebo-controlled trials of the three modern AChE inhibitors (four with donepezil, four with rivastigmine and five with galantamine). Most were designed to demonstrate superiority of the target drug over placebo in cognitive function and a measure of clinicians' impression of change. The consensus view is that this class of drugs offers an average delay in symptom progression of 6 months or more when compared with placebo. Up to 50% of those treated show a four-point or greater improvement over placebo on the ADAS-cog, a scale for cognitive change. Among these responders, about half show an effect size of 7 or more points on the ADAS-cog, at which point improvement is typically obvious to clinicians and carers alike. Studies that also report ADL scores typically show benefits consistent with improvement in cognitive scores. Although the ADL benefits are somewhat smaller, they are likely to be relevant in terms of reduced disability and delayed institutionalization.

In general, AChE inhibitors are well tolerated, with donepezil perhaps better tolerated than others. The most common adverse reactions relate to cholinergic effects on the gastrointestinal tract (nausea, vomiting and diarrhea), with an excess of actively treated patient withdrawals over placebo of approximately 5%.

Data from Canada suggest that institutionalization is responsible for the largest part of dementia costs. Economic predictions suggest that use of donepezil for mild-to-moderate Alzheimer's disease reduces 5-year costs and lessens the time spent in the severe phase of Alzheimer's disease when compared with the alternative of usual care. In US patients with Alzheimer's disease being cared for at home, treatment with donepezil over a 6-month study period did not increase overall direct medical costs. Between four and six patients would need to be treated with donepezil 10 mg once daily over 6 months to achieve in one patient an improvement of 4 points on the ADAS-cog in excess of the response expected by chance.

Routine clinical experience in the 'real world' outside the clinical trial setting indicates that about one half of patients show some cognitive improvement and a minority improve quite markedly. The typical response to an AChE inhibitor in a patient with Alzheimer's disease is subtle but with identifiable improvement within 12 weeks in attentiveness, reduction in apathy or improvement in conversational language and ADL, sufficient to make some difference to those caring for the patient. In addition, patients with behavioral problems often show the most clinically significant benefit, as assessed by carers and formal assessments such as the neuropsychiatric inventory (NPI; see page 56) and its carer distress scale. The Southampton Memory Clinic found that 49% of patients showed improvement from baseline on the NPI; 37% showed an improvement of at least 4 points.

Practical aspects of acetylcholinesterase inhibitor use. Therapy should be initiated once the diagnosis of Alzheimer's disease is likely and there are no contraindications. In the UK, therapy should be introduced by an experienced clinician. Advanced age is not a contraindication. It is usual to withdraw concomitant medication about 3 weeks before initiation of therapy. An electrocardiogram is not routinely necessary but should be performed if there are irregularities in the pulse. Clinical chemistry, including measurement of liver enzymes, should be recorded at baseline and reviewed at 3 months and 1 year.

Evidence of effectiveness is an important determinant for continuation of therapy and should be sought using a standardized scale. Although it was not designed for the purpose, many clinicians find the mini mental state examination (MMSE; see page 52) total score to be an adequate guide to changes in disease severity. Decisions to withdraw a drug because of lack of effect, usually after 12–18 months, can be supported by a decline in the MMSE score of more than 5 points over a year of treatment despite an adequate dose. However, several experts have reported that lack of response to one AChE inhibitor need not imply failure of all these drugs as a class. They therefore suggest an earlier change (perhaps after a few months) to a different drug in this class.

Memantine

Memantine is a derivative of the antiviral drug amantidine, which was unexpectedly found to reduce the symptoms of Parkinson's disease. Like amantidine, memantine is a weak promoter of dopamine release, but it is also a much stronger antagonist of a receptor involved in cell death through a mechanism called excitotoxicity. These receptors are normally activated by the amino acid L-glutamate, which is the major excitatory transmitter in the brain. Receptors stimulated by glutamate are present in several forms; one of which is selectively stimulated by the amino acid analog *N*-methyl-D-aspartate (NMDA) and is known as the NMDA receptor. Memantine is a specific but partial antagonist of the NMDA receptor. When stimulated, NMDA receptors allow calcium to enter the neuron and trigger biochemical changes that underpin the modifications of synaptic function involved in memory and learning. The activity of large cortical pyramidal neurons represents a delicate balance between excitatory (glutamate) and inhibitory (GABA) inputs. Excessive and prolonged stimulation of NMDA receptors disrupts this balance and is highly toxic to neurons (glutamate excitotoxicity). When this stimulation causes neurons to be overloaded with calcium, many calcium-dependent enzymes (proteases) are over-activated and there is excess generation of free radicals. This type of 'glutamate excitotoxicity' is probably involved in cell death after stroke, in poorly controlled epilepsy and in some age-related neurodegenerative diseases like Huntington's disease and Alzheimer's disease.

Memantine is of modest value in the treatment of Parkinson's disease, and this encouraged its use in the treatment of other age-related neurodegenerative conditions since about 1990. Evidence from current randomized clinical trials of memantine in Alzheimer's disease is awaited, but the results of two relevant studies are available. In one Swedish study, 82 patients with severe dementia (MMSE scores < 10 points) received memantine 10 mg per day, while 84 received placebo. Dementia diagnoses included both Alzheimer's disease and vascular dementia but may also have included mixed types. After 12 weeks, care needs were slightly but significantly less in patients taking memantine than in those taking the placebo. In the second study, French patients with vascular dementia (MMSE scores 12–20) were randomly assigned to memantine 20 mg daily or placebo. After 28 weeks, scores on ADAS-cog showed significant advantages of memantine over placebo. At present it is too early to assess the possible role of memantine in the routine treatment of Alzheimer's disease. Memantine therapy is likely to be beneficial in the treatment of vascular dementia. Cerebrovascular pathology is commonplace in late-onset Alzheimer's disease and may be intimately involved in the pathogenesis of amyloid formation.

Encouraging results were reported in conference proceedings in 2002 from at least one adequately sized trial in patients with severe Alzheimer's disease. Those treated with memantine showed negligible progression of their symptom severity over a year of observation, whereas those treated with placebo declined predictably.

Combination treatment

A recent trial showed improvement in dementia symptoms among patients with moderate-to-severe Alzheimer's disease or mixed Alzheimer–vascular dementias when memantine was added to stable treatment with donepezil. This combination therapy with memantine and donepezil (and, by inference, probably other cholinesterase inhibitors) shows potential benefit beyond that of the cholinesterase inhibitor alone.

Treating pain

The World Health Organization recommendations for the treatment of cancer pain are also applicable to dementia (Figure 7.1). Non-opioid (e.g. non-steroidal anti-inflammatory drugs) and opioid analgesics are the cornerstone of pharmacological pain management; tricyclic antidepressants and anticonvulsants are useful adjuvants. These drugs can also be effective when used alone in the treatment of certain types of neuropathic pain; however, care must be taken when using drugs with anticholinergic side effects that might worsen cognitive impairment.

Treating behavioral problems

The non-pharmacological strategies for managing behavioral problems in dementia are discussed in Chapter 6. Table 7.1 lists drugs commonly used to treat behavioral symptoms in dementia. As a general rule, drugs should be used only for serious problems: delusions and hallucinations, risk of injury to self or others, or in the presence of severe and persistent distress. Doses determined in trials to treat schizophrenia do not reliably guide prescribing practice in old people with dementia. In addition to neuroleptic drugs and anticonvulsants (for aggression), antidepressants are often used, though again there is little formal evidence to support their use in patients with dementia.

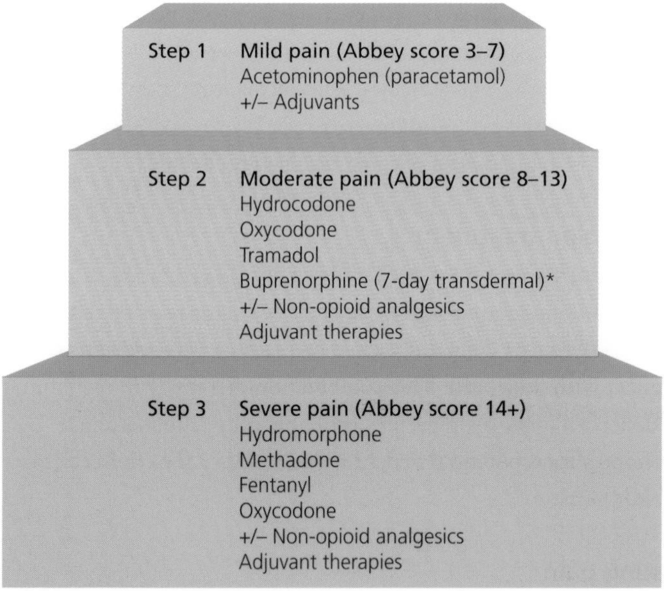

Step 1	**Mild pain (Abbey score 3–7)** Acetominophen (paracetamol) +/– Adjuvants
Step 2	**Moderate pain (Abbey score 8–13)** Hydrocodone Oxycodone Tramadol Buprenorphine (7-day transdermal)* +/– Non-opioid analgesics Adjuvant therapies
Step 3	**Severe pain (Abbey score 14+)** Hydromorphone Methadone Fentanyl Oxycodone +/– Non-opioid analgesics Adjuvant therapies

*In Australia and Europe.
Non-opioid analgesics include non-steroidal anti-inflammatory drugs (NSAIDs).
Adjuvants include massage, transdermal electrical nerve stimulation (TENS) and acupuncture.

Figure 7.1 Good practice stepwise plan for the management of pain in patients with dementia (adapted from the World Health Organization ladder of standard step therapies). The Abbey pain score is illustrated in Table 6.2, page 68.

TABLE 7.1

Drugs used to treat behavioral problems in dementia

Neuroleptics	Non-neuroleptics
• Haloperidol	• Chlormethiazole (not available in the US)
• Quetiapine	• Benzodiazepines
• Olanzapine	• Antidepressants, particularly SSRIs
• Risperidone	• Anticonvulsants, especially valproate
	• Lithium

SSRI, selective serotonin-reuptake inhibitor

Key points – pharmacological treatment

- Treatment frequently provides benefits in terms of mitigation of cognitive decline and ADL and amelioration of neuropsychiatric symptoms.
- The less well-documented but clinically important effects such as the neuropsychiatric benefit and the benefit to caregivers' well-being are of great value in clinical practice.
- Reduction in institutionalization rates following treatment are greater than those seen following care in a stroke unit.
- The economic case remains unproven, but in the absence of an effect on survival, drug costs are likely to be outweighed by delayed institutionalization costs.
- In vascular dementia, the acetyl cholinesterase inhibitors may contribute to improved cognitive performance and improved global function. However, side effects are more common in vascular dementia.
- For patients with more severe Alzheimer's or mixed dementias, the addition of memantine may provide a further improvement in outcome.
- The World Health Organization recommendations for the treatment of cancer pain are also applicable to the treatment of pain in dementia patients; non-opioid and opioid analgesics are the treatment of choice, while tricyclic antidepressants and anticonvulsants are useful adjuvants.
- Drugs should be used for serious psychiatric problems only, such as delusions and hallucinations, risk of injury to self or others, or in the presence of severe and persistent distress.

Key references

Orogozo JM, Rigaud AS, Stoffler A et al. Efficacy and safety of memantine in patients with mild to moderate vascular dementia – a randomized placebo-controlled trial (MMM300). *Stroke* 2002;33: 1834–9.

Rogers SL, Friedhoff LT. Long-term efficacy and safety of donepezil in the treatment of Alzheimer's disease: an interim analysis of the results of a US multicentre open label extension study. *Eur Neuropsychopharmacol* 1998;8:67–75.

Rosler M, Anand R, Cicin-Sain A et al. Efficacy and safety of rivastigmine in patients with Alzheimer's disease: international randomised controlled trial. *BMJ* 1999;318:633–8.

Starr JM, Whalley LJ, Deary IJ. The effects of antihypertensive treatment on cognitive function: results from the HOPE study. *J Am Geriatr Soc* 1996;44:411–15.

Winblatt B, Poritis N. Memantine in severe dementia: results of the M-9-BEST study (benefit and efficacy in severely demented patients during treatment with memantine). *Int J Ger Psychiatr* 1999;14:135–46.

8 Epidemiology of the dementing illnesses

Studying the distribution of an illness within and among populations, and the factors associated with alterations in such distribution, can tell us much about the causes of the illness, and possibly about its prevention.

Prevalence

The prevalence of a particular condition is the proportion or percentage of a population affected by it. Together with consideration of the severity of the condition, it is the appropriate measure for the burden of a disease in a population. Prevalence is determined by both the incidence of a disease (the rate of appearance of new cases) and the duration of illness once it is evident.

The prevalence of dementia is increasing throughout the world, in part because of increased survival after onset of symptoms. With improved nursing care and more widespread use of antibiotics to treat intercurrent infections, individuals now commonly survive 10 years or longer with dementia. This was not always the case – in the 1950s, the pioneering geriatric psychiatrist Sir Martin Roth and colleagues used distinctions in duration of illness to show that dementia differed from other severe psychiatric syndromes, notably depression, in the elderly. At that time, most elderly people hospitalized with dementia in the UK survived for approximately 2 years; those with depression survived longer. The increasing prevalence of dementia that has resulted from longer survival after disease onset has been cited by the late American epidemiologist Ernest Gruenberg as one of several 'failures of success' – a phrase he coined to describe advances in practice that, paradoxically, result in an increased burden of disease. Incidentally, the same unfortunate principle applies to treatments that slow progression (and therefore delay death) in established cases of Alzheimer's disease or other dementias.

Reliable estimation of prevalence depends on accurate identification of cases of the specified condition. For both clinical and epidemiological purposes, the diagnosis of Alzheimer's disease requires both the exclusion of other causes of dementia and the presence of key or characteristic features, as described in Chapter 5. Alzheimer's disease is by far the most common cause of the dementia syndrome in the Western world. With the exception of cerebrovascular disease, which is apparently more common in Japan than elsewhere, other causes are relatively rare and account for only a few percent of cases. Table 8.1 shows the relative frequencies of the various illnesses that underlie prevalent dementia in Europe and North America. It can be seen that dementia often has multiple causes, and the combination of Alzheimer's disease with cerebrovascular disease in particular is more frequent than would be predicted if the two were unrelated. The common concurrence of Alzheimer's and vascular pathology has led to debate concerning the relative frequencies of these two diseases, as investigators tend to give different emphasis to one or the other at diagnosis.

Risk factors for dementia and Alzheimer's disease

A risk factor is an individual characteristic or attribute that is observed to modify the incidence of a condition (and hence, typically, its prevalence). Age is the key risk factor for dementia. The condition is rare in young or middle-aged adults but becomes extremely common in old age. Between the ages of 75 and 80 years (a typical age at death for those who have survived to a nominal retirement age of 65 years), 10% of people will typically develop dementia. Yet, contrary to popular belief reflected in the term 'senility' or 'senile dementia', age itself is

TABLE 8.1

Causes of dementia

- Alzheimer's disease (50%)
- Mixed Alzheimer–vascular diseases (20%)
- Cerebrovascular disease (10%)
- Lewy body dementia (10%)
- 'Reversible' causes* (5%)
- Unknown cause (5%)

*See Table 3.2, page 37.

not a cause of dementia. Many very old people have intact cognition ('successful aging' – see pages 27 and 28). This observation supports the principle that association does not imply cause. The 'cognitive reserve' hypothesis is widely regarded as being responsible for the observation that Alzheimer's disease is less common in those with greater educational or occupational attainment. Figure 8.1a depicts identical neurodegenerative processes in two individuals with different cognitive capacities in early life. Individual (i) starts with less cerebral reserve, so his trajectory crosses the symptom threshold a few years earlier (i.e. this person experiences earlier onset and higher age-specific risk of Alzheimer's disease). Figure 8.1b shows the effect of various isoforms of apolipoprotein E, a cholesterol transport protein with normal variants that predict different onsets and age-specific risks for Alzheimer's disease (see Chapter 9). These variants also predict the trajectory in middle age of cognitive abilities or of early metabolic and anatomic brain features predicted by this model of Alzheimer's disease. Figure 8.1c suggests the possible effects of environmental risk or protective factors that can accelerate or retard the underlying process, resulting in disease onset earlier or later than otherwise expected (exaggerated or attenuated age-specific risk).

Sex. All prevalence studies show that women are more often affected by dementia than are men. Typically, health services treat twice as many women as men with dementia. This contrast is explained only partly by the longer life expectancy of women because, even when this is taken into account, a slight excess of incidence is still evident in women. Recent studies from Europe and the USA have shown that this small increase reflects a strong disproportion in the incidence of Alzheimer's disease among women after 85 years of age. With increasing life expectancy, one may therefore expect a still greater excess of women with Alzheimer's disease. Some of this excess may be caused by impairment of neuronal function and neuronal protective mechanisms with estrogen depletion after menopause. Social factors (e.g. widowhood) may also exacerbate the apparent disability associated with dementia in older women. Social and biological aging processes probably act together to increase the burden of disability in

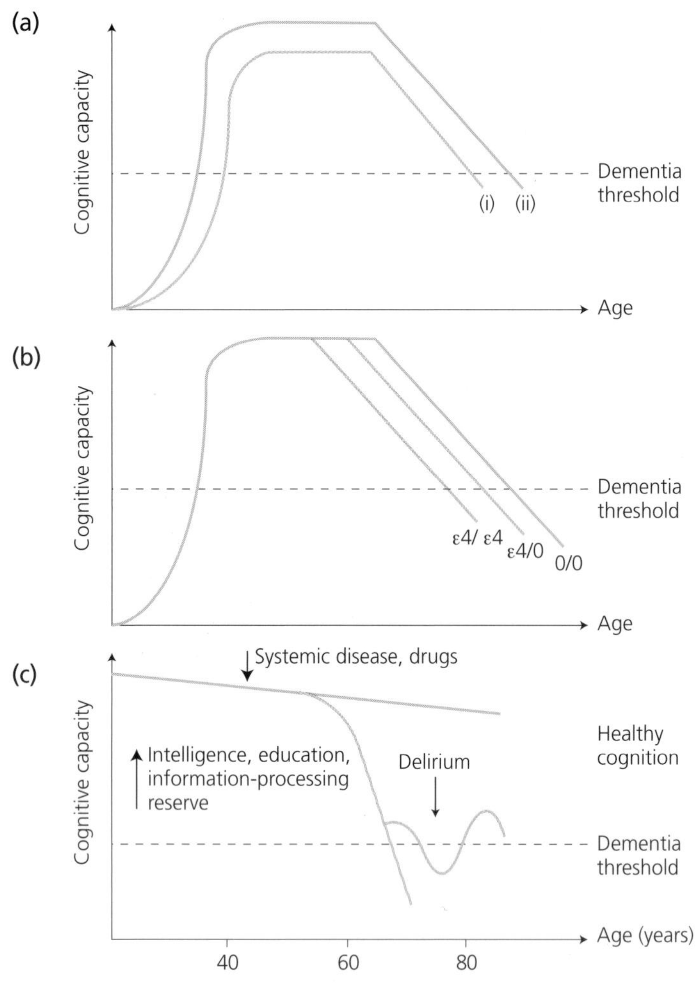

Figure 8.1 (a) Outcome of identical neurodegenerative processes in two individuals with substantially different cognitive capacities in early life. Individual (i) starts with less cerebral reserve than (ii) and so experiences earlier onset of Alzheimer's disease. (b) Example of a genetic risk factor: ε4 is a variant of the apolipoprotein E allele (see Chapter 9); two copies increase the risk of early-onset Alzheimer's disease; one copy has less effect. (c) Possible effects of environmental risk or protective factors that can accelerate or retard the underlying process, resulting in disease onset earlier or later than otherwise expected.

elderly women for whom the added burden of age-related cognitive impairment leads to decompensation of adaptive processes.

Family history. Individuals whose first-degree relatives (parents, siblings) have Alzheimer's disease show an approximate threefold increased risk of developing Alzheimer's disease compared with those who lack such a family history. This increase holds across the spectrum of ages. Thus, person A who has an affected sibling may have three times the risk of person B who does not, whether both A and B are aged 65 or 85 years; however, the absolute risks at the later age are much higher: an 85-year-old person without a family history has a higher risk than a 65-year-old with an affected relative.

Although Alzheimer's disease tends to run in families, the majority of present-day patients with Alzheimer's disease do not in fact have an affected relative. This is because a familial predisposition to Alzheimer's disease is expressed mainly in relatives of very old age. Probably, fewer than half of predisposed individuals develop the disease before 85 years of age. Therefore, the absence of a family history may simply reflect the absence of sufficient numbers of very old relatives to reveal the familial tendency toward the disease. The familial aggregation of Alzheimer's disease may reflect shared cultural or environmental background as well as genes, although the latter are clearly important. Hypotheses about the genetic causes of Alzheimer's disease are discussed in Chapter 9.

Race and geography. A higher prevalence of vascular dementia among African-Americans is usually attributed to the higher prevalence of cardiovascular risk factors and lower socioeconomic status of this vulnerable group. Specifically, about 25% of Americans have hypertension, but the age-adjusted prevalence of hypertension among African-Americans compared with white Americans is about 33%.

Large differences in the proportion of dementia attributable to vascular dementia are reported between Asia and Europe. In Europe, there are about 17 patients with Alzheimer's disease for every 10 with mixed or vascular dementia; by contrast, in Japan the diagnosis of vascular dementia is more common. Comparisons between ethnically homogeneous Japanese populations in Japan, Hawaii and Washington

State in the USA suggest that these contrasts may be attributed largely to cultural or environmental variation. As populations have migrated from Japan to Hawaii or to the US mainland, the ratio of Alzheimer cases to vascular cases has approximated to that seen in other American populations.

Vascular pathology. Vascular lesions can exaggerate the clinical effects of Alzheimer pathology. In this sense, strokes and other vascular changes may act as 'risk factors' for the onset of dementia in those developing Alzheimer's disease. Important risk factors for such vascular pathology, and indeed for vascular dementia, include:

- poorly controlled hypertension
- diabetes mellitus
- hyperhomocysteinemia
- hyperlipidemias
- smoking
- various indices of an individual's general tendency towards atherosclerosis.

Alcohol consumption. There are conflicting views on whether moderate alcohol consumption increases the risk of dementia, or on whether one type of alcoholic beverage has advantages over another in terms of risk reduction. There is no doubt, however, that continued excessive alcohol use is harmful, and that the aging brain is particularly vulnerable to these effects. Currently, moderate alcohol consumption over 65 years of age (fewer than 15 standard alcoholic drinks per week among men, fewer among women) is not believed to increase dementia risk. In fact, light alcohol intake (fewer than seven standard drinks per week) appears to be associated with a lower risk of dementia and Alzheimer's disease. The mechanism of the protective action of low alcohol intake is not understood but at least one intriguing report has suggested that regular consumption of red wine is associated with a reduced risk of Alzheimer's disease. Red wine contains antioxidant flavonoids that, together with antioxidant vitamins, may have direct neuroprotective effects. Red wine is thought also to protect against cardiovascular disease, and therefore perhaps cerebrovascular disease, and it may reduce the risk of Alzheimer's disease by attenuating the influence of these known risk factors.

Dietary risk factors. Among environmental influences, dietary variation may be an important modifier of risk for dementia. Many reports suggest inverse relationships between intake of foods such a fruit and vegetables (rich sources of antioxidants and other micronutrients) and risk of Alzheimer's disease; however, in the face of some contrary findings, no consensus exists on their relative importance. The controversy may reflect that consumption of many foodstuffs is highly inter-related; the unreliability of dietary self-reports in the presence of cognitive impairment; or the genetic heterogeneity between samples. Among foodstuffs, a case is made for a role of low dietary intake of omega-3 polyunsaturated fatty acids as a risk factor for age-related cognitive decline, although not all reports support this hypothesis.

Homocysteine. The Framingham follow-up study has provided compelling evidence that increased plasma homocysteine is a relevant risk factor for Alzheimer's disease, and a substantial body of evidence now supports an inverse relationship between plasma homocysteine and cognitive function in late life. Current estimates suggest that 8–10% of age-related cognitive variation can be attributed to homocysteine. Figure 8.2 shows the cumulative incidence of dementia in Framingham subjects in the highest quartile of plasma homocysteine (> 13.2 μmol/L). Possible mechanisms to explain the increased dementia risk linked to homocysteine include its known oxidative potential to damage neuronal membranes and DNA and its capacity to sensitize neurons to the harmful effects of amyloid.

Folic acid and vitamin B_{12} supplementation can lower homocysteine by 25–35% in hyperhomocysteinemia. The extent of reduction is partly modified by a polymorphism in the methylenetetrahydrofolate reductase (MTHFR) gene and by the dose of folate. Clinical trials to prevent or postpone dementia onset in at-risk individuals by lowering plasma homocysteine levels suggest that mitigation of hyperhomocysteinemia can slow cognitive aging, but as yet it is uncertain whether the intervention will delay or even prevent dementia onset.

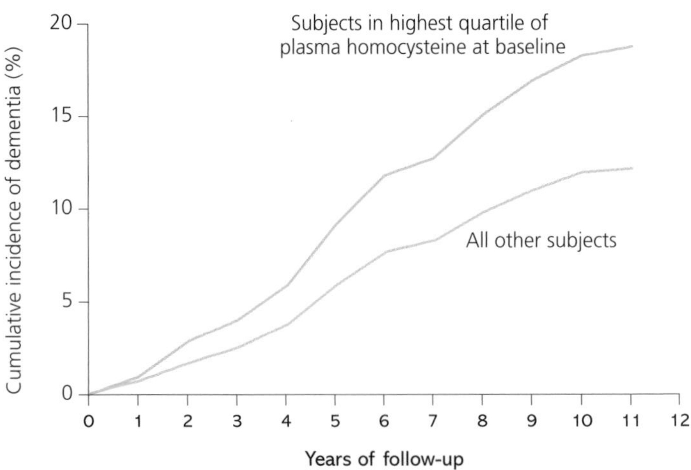

Figure 8.2 Cumulative incidence of dementia in subjects in the highest quartile of plasma homocysteine (> 13.2 μmol/L). Adapted from Seshadri et al. 2002.

Other risk and possible protective factors for Alzheimer's disease. It is clear that not all people experience a similarly increased risk of dementia as they age. For example, those who have suffered moderate-to-severe head injury, sufficient to cause more than an hour's loss of consciousness or amnesia, are probably at increased risk. By contrast, people of higher intelligence or greater educational attainment are at reduced risk. The reasons for this are incompletely understood, but a reasonable explanation portrays Alzheimer's disease as a chronic neurodegenerative process that begins many years before the onset of dementia itself (Figures 3.1 [page 31] and 8.1). It includes a long latent stage that may last for several decades, as well as a prodromal phase that probably accounts for much, but certainly not all, of the phenomenon of mild age-related cognitive decline. Those with more 'cerebral reserve' can tolerate more neurodegeneration before symptoms of dementia become evident. The hypothetical concept of 'cerebral reserve' may explain why low educational level so often appears as a risk factor for Alzheimer's disease. In most cultures, educational attainment is highly correlated with intelligence and with synaptic density. The few studies that have attempted to separate the highly correlated attributes of intelligence and education suggest that the former 'drives' the relationship between education and the risk of Alzheimer's disease, though this remains controversial.

Other environmental influences may also slow the progression of the Alzheimer's process. Notably, these influences are thought to act principally in the latent or prodromal states of this process, so that their effect is a delay in the age at which dementia symptoms appear. The benefit of the several factors that may achieve such delay seems to be limited to a critical time window; that is, the effect may disappear a variable number of years before dementia symptoms would otherwise occur. There is an emerging consensus that four main groups of factors, each determined by careful epidemiological study, have sufficient potential to help retain cognitive function in old age and may delay dementia onset:

- control of vascular risk factors
- physical activity
- continuing social and intellectual engagement
- a healthy, well-balanced, nutrient-dense but energy-poor diet.

Among several other possible protective influences, the following are now thought to be promising.

- Hormone replacement therapy among postmenopausal women. However, there is no evidence for benefit of this intervention within the 10 years before onset of dementia symptoms.
- Sustained use of non-steroidal anti-inflammatory drugs. Here the benefit seems to disappear 2 or 3 years before onset of dementia. The 'protective' influence of these drugs also seems to disappear after about 80 years of age. The available evidence suggests that full anti-inflammatory doses do not offer any greater protective effect than low analgesic doses.
- Antioxidant vitamin supplements. Antioxidants are the only interventions shown in large trials to produce a disease-modifying effect after dementia symptoms are evident, and their benefits for prevention may be sustained longer than the other interventions described here. More recent data have shown, however, that these treatments (e.g. high-dose vitamin E) are not without risks of their own.

Note that none of these interventions has yet been demonstrated to be effective in randomized trials, so that their benefits are not proven.

Risk factors for other types of dementia. Much less is known about the epidemiology of other rarer causes of dementia than about the epidemiology of Alzheimer's disease and vascular dementia. With the possible exception of Lewy body dementia (an entity that borders controversially with Alzheimer's disease in some cases and with Parkinson's disease in others), none of these rarer conditions accounts for more than a few percent of dementia cases. As is true of Alzheimer's disease, their incidence increases among the very old. Their relationship to age is much weaker, however, than that of Alzheimer's disease. As a result, the older the population, the greater the relative frequency of Alzheimer's disease as a cause of dementia. Figure 8.3 shows the increase with age in the proportion of dementia caused by Alzheimer's

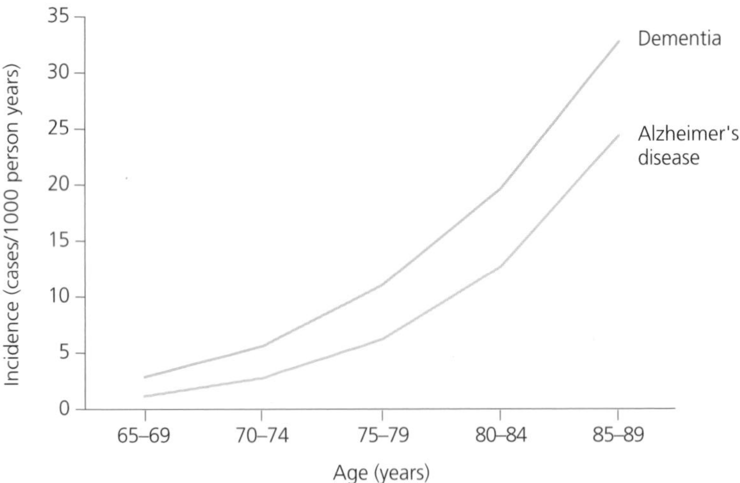

Figure 8.3 The age-specific incidence of moderate-to-severe dementia and Alzheimer's disease in Europe and the USA (adapted from Jorm and Jolley 1998). The figure suggests a growth with age that is more or less exponential between the ages of 65 and 85, with the rate doubling every 5 years. Thereafter, the increase may slow somewhat. If milder cases are included, the rates are approximately double those depicted.

disease. You can see that, at 65 years of age, Alzheimer's disease typically represents about half of all dementias, but by 85 years the proportion has increased to well over three-quarters. Many people now live to 85 years, so the greatest public health concern is Alzheimer's disease.

Key points – epidemiology of the dementing illnesses

- Alzheimer's disease is by far the commonest form of dementia throughout the world. In some less developed areas, vascular and reversible ('treatable') types of dementia may be somewhat more frequent.
- Race and geography contribute to differences in the incidence of dementia, suggesting that environmental factors – possibly nutritional – may be important.
- Age is the most important risk factor for Alzheimer's disease. Family history, cerebrovascular disease and hyperhomocysteinemia are relevant but less important than age.
- Control of vascular risk factors, physical activity, maintenance of social and intellectual engagement and a balanced diet are important in old age and may slow dementia onset.
- Some medicines and nutrients such as antioxidant vitamin supplements may delay the onset of Alzheimer's disease; other possible protective influences include non-steroidal anti-inflammatory drugs and hormone replacement therapy (when used in the decades after menopause).

Key references

Christensen H, Korten AE, Jorm AF et al. Education and decline in cognitive performance: compensatory but not protective. *Int J Geriatr Psychiatry* 1997;12:323–30.

Gao S, Hendrie HC, Hall KS, Hui S. The relationships between age, sex, and the incidence of dementia and Alzheimer disease: a meta-analysis. *Arch Gen Psychiatry* 1998;55: 809–15.

Jorm AF, Jolley D. The incidence of dementia: a meta-analysis. *Neurology* 1998;51:728–33.

Khachaturian ZS, Petersen RC, Gauthier S et al. A roadmap for the prevention of dementia: the inaugural Leon Thal Symposium. *Alzheimers Dement* 2008;4:156–63.

Letenneur L. Risk of dementia and alcohol and wine consumption: a review of recent results. *Biol Res* 2004;37:189–93.

Luchsinger JA, Mayeux R. Dietary factors and Alzheimer's disease. *Lancet Neurol* 2004;3:579–87.

Ott A, Stolk RP, van Harskamp F et al. Diabetes mellitus and the risk of dementia. The Rotterdam Study. *Neurology* 1999;53:1937–42.

Plassman BL, Havlik RJ, Steffens DC et al. Documented head injury in early adulthood and risk of Alzheimer's disease and other dementias. *Neurology* 2000:55: 1158–66.

Prince MJ, Bird AS, Blizzard RA, Mann AH. Is the cognitive function of older patients affected by antihypertensive treatment? Results from 54 months of the Medical Research Council's trial of hypertension in older adults. *BMJ* 1996;312:801–5.

Seshadri S, Beiser A, Selhub et al. Plasma homocysteine as a risk factor for dementia and Alzheimer's disease. *N Engl J Med* 2002;346:476–83.

Szekely CA, Green RC, Breitner JC et al. No advantage of A beta 42-lowering NSAIDs for prevention of Alzheimer dementia in six pooled cohort studies. *Neurology* 2008;70: 2291–8.

Zandi PP, Carlson MC, Plassman BL et al. Hormone replacement therapy and incidence of Alzheimer disease in older women. The Cache County Study. *JAMA* 2002;288:1–7.

9 Hypotheses on the causes of Alzheimer's disease

Genetics

For decades it was thought that rare, early-onset variants of Alzheimer's disease were 'familial' and probably genetic, while the common, later-onset types were 'sporadic'. The familial forms most often showed the characteristics that about half of the offspring of a given case would themselves develop Alzheimer's disease. Males and females appeared equally vulnerable. An example pedigree of this type is shown in Figure 9.1. The usual explanation for such familial aggregation is that

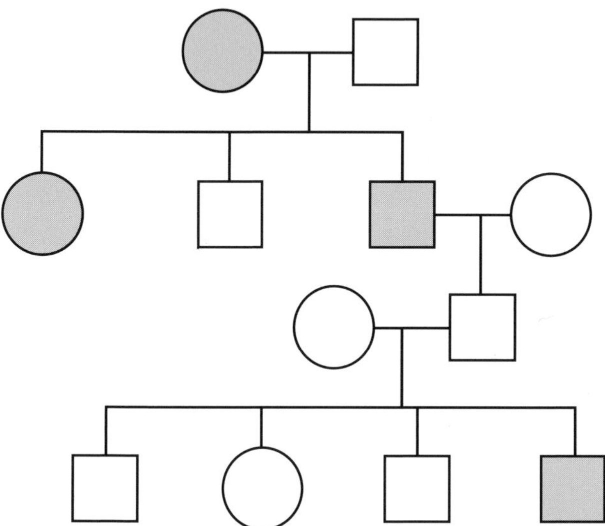

Figure 9.1 A pedigree showing the distribution of Alzheimer's disease cases (filled symbols) among male (squares) and female (circles) members of successive generations. Both sexes are affected at similar rates, and there is no preferential transmission from fathers or mothers. About one-half of the offspring of each case (and thus about one-half of the brothers or sisters of any affected individual) will themselves develop the disease.

the predisposition to disease is transmitted by a single copy of a defective gene located on one of the 22 autosomal chromosomes.

Not all cases of early-onset (< 65 years) Alzheimer's disease show the sort of familial aggregation seen in Figure 9.1, but about half do. In the past 10 years, mutations at three genes have been found to provoke this sort of early-onset familial Alzheimer's disease. These genes probably account for between one-third and one-half of pedigrees like those in Figure 9.1. The remainder are presumably caused by other genes.

The first discovered 'Alzheimer's gene' is in the Down's syndrome region of chromosome 21 and encodes a lengthy protein molecule, the amyloid precursor protein (APP), which can be cleaved near its N-terminus to yield the Aβ peptide. The precise functions of APP are still being investigated, but the protein is known to span the neuronal membrane, having a long cytoplasmic domain, a short and lipophilic transmembrane domain and a relatively short extracellular domain. Figure 9.2 shows how APP spans the membrane. The Aβ fragment resides at the junction of the transmembrane and extracellular domains. Several different point mutations in or adjoining the coding region for the Aβ fragment are now known to provoke the Alzheimer's disease phenotype. A number of other nearby mutations appear to be harmless. The critical role of the pathogenic mutations is to promote cleavage patterns that produce intact Aβ peptide. The inevitable appearance of Alzheimer's disease in individuals with pathogenic APP mutations is some of the strongest evidence for the role of Aβ in the causal pathway for Alzheimer's disease.

The two other known 'Alzheimer's genes' are mutations of novel proteins called 'presenilins', so-called because they are subject to rare mutations that can provoke early-onset ('presenile') familial Alzheimer's disease. The two genes, *PSEN1* (also known as *PS1)* and *PSEN2* (also known as *PS2)* on chromosomes 14 and 1, respectively, are strongly homologous and are probably descendants of a single progenitor gene. Most *PSEN1* mutations cause Alzheimer's disease with an even earlier-onset characteristic (usually in the forties) than is seen with the disease-provoking APP mutations. *PSEN2* mutations have a more variable effect, provoking onsets in the fifties to seventies. Notably, both

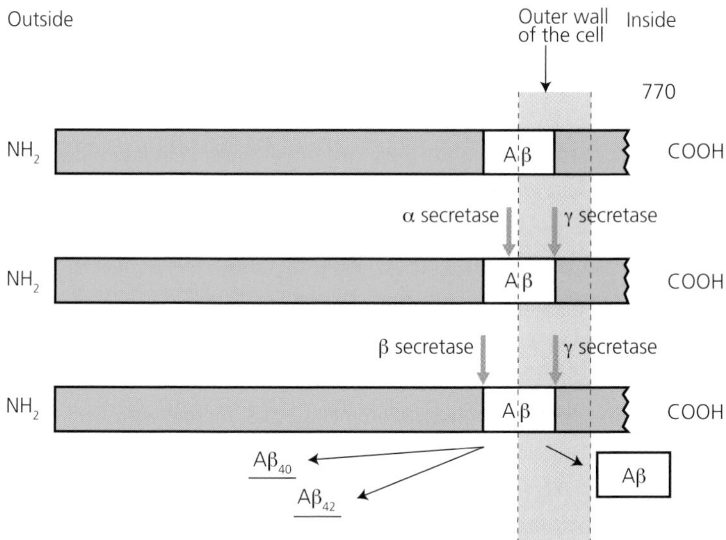

Figure 9.2 The amyloid precursor protein (APP) embedded in a neuronal membrane. The critical Aβ fragment is at the junction of the transmembrane domain of the molecule and its extracellular domain. Three different enzymes are thought to cleave APP in different ways.

presenilin-1 and presenilin-2 are believed to play an important role in the processing of APP and in amyloidogenesis. Their discovery has only served to strengthen support for the importance of the role of Aβ in Alzheimer's disease pathogenesis – even though the exact role of Aβ remains controversial. There is growing evidence to support the possibility that the γ secretase complex (see Figure 9.2) includes presenilin-1.

While these three genes provide important clues to the causal mechanisms of Alzheimer's disease, they are exceedingly rare and therefore are not important causes of Alzheimer's disease (a very common illness). Probably no more than 10% of presenile Alzheimer's disease results from these mutations, and the figure is much smaller (< 1%) for Alzheimer's disease overall. Most Alzheimer's disease occurs in later life and has a much less distinctive pattern of familial aggregation.

The evidence for genetic causes of Alzheimer's disease extends well beyond the phenomena of the rare, early-onset familial variants. Familial aggregation in Alzheimer's disease is strong, even when onset is (typically) late. There are problems here in discerning the true extent of familial aggregation: when the 'fore-ordained' onset is in late old age, many predisposed relatives will die of other unrelated causes before expressing their predisposition by developing Alzheimer's disease. This problem may be dealt with by using survival analysis, a statistical approach that attempts to adjust for the effects of mortality from other causes by considering only those relatives who have survived to a particular age. Survival analyses have shown, for instance, that a first-degree relative (parent, sibling or offspring) of someone with well-diagnosed Alzheimer's disease will him/herself have a 40–50% chance of developing Alzheimer's disease if he or she lives beyond 90 years of age. Similar methods suggest that the comparable risk among first-degree relatives of unaffected population 'control' subjects is lower. Both figures are probably underestimates, reflecting difficulty in ascertainment of dementia in elderly relatives, many of whom are long deceased. The risk to first-degree relatives of patients with Alzheimer's disease is increased about threefold.

How much of this risk is genetic and how much is acquired through shared environment? Answers to this sort of question come from the study of twin pairs. Although twins are born at the same time and are typically reared in circumstances where they share many of their early environmental influences, monozygotic (MZ) and dizygotic (DZ) twin pairs differ importantly in their biology. Twin studies compare the degree of similarity within MZ and DZ pairs, typically also comparing this with similarity among random pairings of unrelated individuals. Substantial differences in the within-pair similarity between MZ and DZ pairs provides strong evidence that genes are responsible for the trait being measured. If that trait is the tendency towards development of a condition such as Alzheimer's disease, then there will be differences in the proportions of twin pairs in which both members have the disease (concordant pairs) as opposed to those in which only one is affected (discordant pairs). Particularly when the population rates of a disease are known (i.e. the chance that another individual chosen at random will have the disease), statistical techniques can be used to estimate the degree to which the predisposition to the disease is inherited, as well as the degree to which shared environmental influences contribute to a general tendency toward disease concordance in both types of twins. Thus, the relative contributions of genes, shared environmental influences, and other unique environmental influences (the residual after the first two are considered) can be estimated from twin studies. This technique can also provide important information to guide the search for predisposing genes (when their influence is strong) and for environmental risk factors.

Four published twin studies of Alzheimer's disease all point to an important role for genes in determining susceptibility to Alzheimer's disease. One study in relatively young men suggested that the influence of genes was relatively modest (accounting for about one-third of the population's variation in risk). However, the relative influences of genes and environmental factors does not remain constant as people age: genes typically predispose to the development of Alzheimer's disease in late old age, while environmental factors may modify the risk at earlier ages. Thus, the three other studies, all conducted in older cohorts, provide more meaningful estimates. They suggest that genes account for 50–75% of the population's variation in risk of Alzheimer's disease.

What might these genes be? It is certain that, unlike the mutations at APP or the presenilins, they are not potent enough to assure the development of Alzheimer's disease in virtually all carriers (i.e. they are not sufficient to provoke the phenotype). It is less clear whether one gene, or one of several genes, may be necessary for the development of the Alzheimer's disease phenotype. If so, then presumably some proportion of the population would lack the required gene or genes, and would not be susceptible to Alzheimer's disease. For the remainder, it is likely that several genes can modify an individual's risk of Alzheimer's disease, primarily by altering the age at which one is predisposed to develop the disease. The best known of these is *APOE*, the polymorphic genetic locus for the cholesterol transport protein, apolipoprotein E (apoE). ApoE is uniquely important among the family of lipoprotein fat transporters for brain development and repair. It is produced in the brain, although much more is made in the liver. The protein exists in three common isoforms: apoE2, apoE3 and apoE4. These variants are encoded by three different alleles (normal variations) of the *APOE* gene. The *APOE* system is similar to the well-known ABO family of blood groups. The alleles at *APOE* are called *APOE* ε2, ε3 and ε4. As in the ABO system, each person inherits one of these alleles from each parent. Thus, there are six possible genotypes: ε2/ε2, ε2/ ε3, ε2/ ε4, ε3/ε3, ε3/ε4 and ε4/ε4. These occur in frequencies that are predicted by the frequency of the three alleles. The ε2 allele is relatively rare; ε4 is somewhat more common; but ε3 is found on almost 78% of all chromosomes (Table 9.1).

The *APOE* system is the strongest known genetic determinant of susceptibility to late-onset Alzheimer's disease, but it is important to note that many people with even the risky ε4/ε4 genotype will not

TABLE 9.1

The APOE system and risk for Alzheimer's disease

Allele	Frequency (%)	Genotype	Frequency (%)	Implications for Alzheimer's disease
ε2	7	ε2/ε2	0.5	Not known
ε3	78	ε2/ε3	11	Probably later onset, reduced risk
ε4	15	ε2/ε4	2.0	Probably comparable with ε3/ε3
		ε3/ε3	61	Reference standard for this table
		ε3/ε4	23.5	Earlier onset, about threefold increased risk compared with ε3/ε3
		ε4/ε4	2.0	Much earlier onset; risk vs ε3/ε3 increased many-fold, depending on age

develop the disease even if they live to be 100. In animal models, *APOE* genotype predicts response to brain injury. Possession of the ε4 allele has been associated with less efficient acquisition of exploratory behaviors in young mice. There is also evidence from similar studies that the richness of synaptic development and dendritic outgrowth is reduced in transgenic mice with substitution of a human ε4 allele. Finally, inheritance of the ε4 allele has been associated with slower recovery of mental ability after head injury.

The proportion of the total genetic influence on Alzheimer's disease mediated by *APOE* remains controversial. Most studies suggest that the relative risk with the ε4/ε4 genotype (compared with the common ε3/ε3 type) is between 12 and 20, while that with the ε3/ε4 genotype is between 2 and 4. Since about 2% of individuals bear the former and 24% the latter genotype, one may calculate population attributable risk for these genotypes (and thus for the ε4 allele altogether). Approached this way, it seems that ε4 may account for 50% of population variation in the risk of Alzheimer's disease. It is worth noting, however, that this estimate declines substantially after 85 years of age when Alzheimer's disease is most common.

There are numerous other candidate genes that might explain the remaining genetic risk of Alzheimer's disease. Because these are all almost certainly weaker than *APOE*, they will be harder to detect. Correspondingly larger and more powerful experiments will therefore be needed to show their effect. Smaller underpowered experiments will predictably produce variable results – just as has been seen to date. More powerful family-based association methods, sib-pair linkage methods or genome-wide association studies may offer the solution to this conundrum, and massive new studies of this type are under way.

As a final caveat we note that inheritance does not equal fate, particularly where relatively weak genes are concerned. The twin studies suggest that about one-third of the population's variation in Alzheimer's disease risk is environmental in origin. In Chapter 8 we discussed some of the environmental factors that may underlie this finding, several of which may suggest new roads to the prevention of Alzheimer's disease.

The free-radical/inflammatory hypothesis of Alzheimer's disease

The association between Alzheimer's disease and aging has suggested that biological hypotheses of aging may be relevant to the causes of Alzheimer's disease. The major theories of aging include the free-radical hypothesis, which can also involve mechanisms of innate immunity and inflammation, as follows.

It is well known that Aβ can have a direct neurotoxic effect that is probably mediated by oxidative mechanisms. For example, β-amyloid can activate neuronal membrane oxidation and so generate free radicals. Aβ also appears to damage vascular endothelium. Figure 9.3 shows how β-amyloid that is released from APP can also bind to a large cell-surface molecule called the receptor for advanced glycation endproducts (RAGE). Interaction between β-amyloid and cerebral vessel walls probably disturbs cellular function, and may damage intracellular proteins. In addition to both of these toxic effects, Aβ fibrils appear to

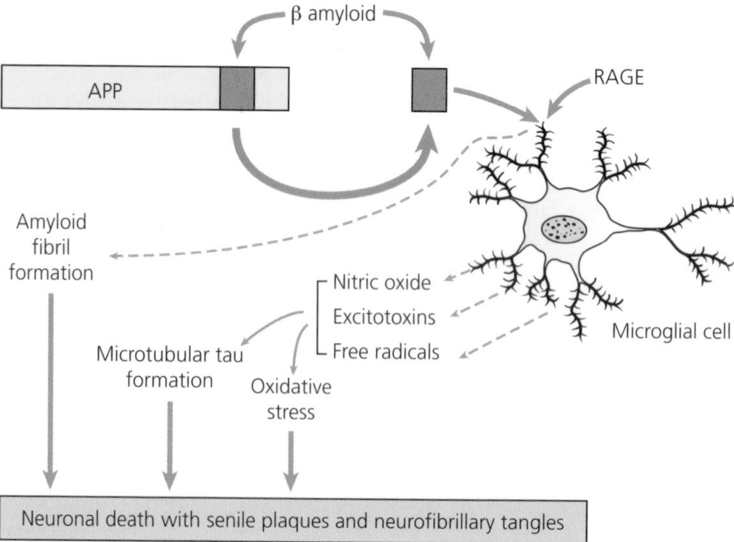

Figure 9.3 Release of β-amyloid from APP to bind at the receptor for advanced glycation endproducts (RAGE) leads to amyloid fibril formation, oxidative stress, then neuronal death with senile plaques and neurofibrillary tangles.

stimulate microglia to produce and release a number of pro-inflammatory and pro-oxidant cytokines, as well as several reactive oxygen species (ROS), into the nearby environment (so-called 'paracrine release'). Activated microglia are commonly seen near amyloid plaques, although it is not clear that they are activated by the plaques themselves. It is equally plausible that plaques arise in areas of higher concentration of fibrillar Aβ oligomers, which are the true stimulus to microglial activation.

The exact role of free-radical formation in these processes is interesting but not certain. Oxidative damage to neurons in Alzheimer's disease is as likely be a consequence of neuronal damage as a cause of it. The location of the gene coding for the enzyme superoxide dismutase 1 (*SOD1*) within the 'Down's syndrome region' of chromosome 21 suggested a reason for the common occurrence of Alzheimer's disease in Down's syndrome. Cultured neurons from Down's syndrome fetuses have also been found to generate increased amounts of ROS, presumably leading to neuronal death by apoptosis. These ROS-mediated mechanisms may therefore account for both the abnormal brain development in Down's syndrome and, later, to the early onset of Alzheimer's disease.

The paracrine release by microglia of pro-inflammatory and pro-oxidant molecular species may be a principal target of non-steroidal anti-inflammatory drugs (NSAIDs) which numerous observational studies have shown to delay the onset of Alzheimer's disease. The primary biological activity of NSAIDs is to block the action of cyclooxygenase (COX) enzymes responsible for the oxidation of cell membrane arachidonic acid to prostaglandins, which stimulate downstream production of other molecular species that promote the secretion of pro-oxidant and pro-inflammatory cytokines. Thus, the 'amyloid toxicity' hypothesis of Alzheimer's disease,' the 'free-radical theory of aging,' and the role of inflammation and innate immunity are not mutually incompatible; instead they may converge to account for much Alzheimer-type degeneration in neurons. Taken together, these observations suggest that future studies will continue to support the neurotoxic effects of β-amyloid and may point to therapeutic strategies, such as vitamin E supplements, that seek both to preserve cerebrovascular endothelium and to reduce the neurotoxic effects of pro-oxidative cytokines.

Tau protein, neurofibrillary tangles and Alzheimer's disease

The neuropathology of Alzheimer's disease includes the formation of neurofibrillary tangles (NFTs) and it is these lesions, rather than amyloid plaques, that appear to correlate more closely with the appearance of dementia symptoms. The appearance of NFTs characteristically begins in the entorhinal cortex in the anteromesial temporal lobes. As the disease progresses, tangles appear elsewhere in temporal lobe structures, particularly in the CA-1 region critical for memory formation, and in the superior temporal gyrus. Further progression results in the appearance of NFTs in the angular gyrus and temporo-parietal region which, together with the superior temporal gyrus, are essential for language function. Later, more generalized involvement of the parietal lobes and frontal cortex accounts for the characteristic apraxia and agnosia that characterize Alzheimer's dementia. Thus, the extent and distribution of NFTs is closely correlated with both the degree of dementia and its characteristic cascade of clinical features. It is therefore difficult to account for the symptoms of Alzheimer's disease using the 'amyloid toxicity hypothesis' alone, but it is also true that we currently have no explanation for the disease's characteristic progression of NFT pathology.

The NFTs contain paired helical filaments (PHFs) that are composed of the microtubule-associated protein (MAP) tau in an abnormally phosphorylated state. Tau is present throughout nervous tissue, and at least six different splice variants of it are present in adult brain, all derived by differential processing of a single gene product. All six adult brain isoforms of tau are hyperphosphorylated in Alzheimer's disease. In health, tau proteins (together with tubulin) promote polymerization of microtubules. When tau is hyperphosphorylated, however, such polymerization does not occur; instead tau aggregates into the PHFs that form the characteristic NFTs of Alzheimer's disease.

NFTs have proven difficult to study, mostly because of their relative insolubility. This same characteristic allows the NFT to survive after the death of a neuron, giving rise to 'tombstone' or 'ghost' tangles. Because the hyperphosphorylation of tau protein appears to be a key step in the initiation of other molecular pathological events that produce the characteristic neurodegenerative changes of Alzheimer's disease, the molecular mechanisms of tau phosphorylation and aggregation are now being investigated as a potential therapeutic target for the development of drugs to prevent Alzheimer's disease.

Key points – hypotheses on the causes of Alzheimer's disease

- Genetic factors are relevant to all forms of Alzheimer's disease, irrespective of age at onset or family history.
- In rare familial forms of early-onset dementia, faulty genes are involved in about one-fifth of cases. These code for a cellular adhesion molecule (amyloid precursor protein, APP) or for molecules involved in APP processing (presenilins).
- Population studies indicate that a substantial part – perhaps 50–75% – of the risk of late-onset Alzheimer's disease is influenced by genetic factors.
- Many genetic risk factors are unidentified. Polymorphisms in the APOE gene that encodes the lipid transport protein apolipoprotein E may determine timing of the onset of Alzheimer's disease but do not appear to cause it directly.
- Environmental influences account for at least 25% of a person's predisposition to Alzheimer's disease, probably more.
- Neuronal death in Alzheimer's disease is associated with cleavage of the Aβ fragment from the amyloid precursor protein. Aβ aggregates have direct toxic effects on neurons but, perhaps more importantly, they damage vascular endothelium and stimulate the activation of microglial cells that release of pro-oxidative cytokines.
- The link between the effects of Aβ and the degeneration of synapses and neurons is not known, but the aggregation of hyperphosphorylated tau protein into paired helical filaments and neurofibrillary tangles is a more direct correlate of cognitive dysfunction than is density of amyloid plaques.

Key references

Athan ES, Williamson J, Ciappa A et al. A founder mutation in presenilin 1 causing early-onset Alzheimer disease in unrelated Caribbean Hispanic families. *JAMA* 2001; 286:2257–63.

Bertram L, Lange C, Mullin K et al. Genome-wide association analysis reveals putative Alzheimer's disease susceptibility loci in addition to APOE. *Am J Hum Genet* 2008;83:623–32.

Bertram L, Tanzi RE. Thirty years of Alzheimer's disease genetics: the implications of systematic meta-analyses. *Nat Rev Neurosci* 2008;9:768–78.

den Heijer T, Launer LJ, Prins ND et al. Association between blood pressure, white matter lesions, and atrophy of the medial temporal lobe. *Neurology* 2005;64:263–7.

Farris W, Mansourian S, Leissring MA et al. Partial loss-of-function mutations in insulin-degrading enzyme that induce diabetes also impair degradation of amyloid beta-protein. *Am J Pathol* 2004;164: 1425–34.

Fernández JA, Rojo L, Kuljis RO, Maccioni RB. The damage signals hypothesis of Alzheimer's disease pathogenesis. *J Alzheimers Dis* 2008;14:329–33.

Fratiglioni L, Wang HX. Smoking and Parkinson's and Alzheimer's disease: review of the epidemiological studies. *Behav Brain Res* 2000; 113:117–20.

Goedert M. Tau protein and the neurofibrillary pathology of Alzheimer's disease. *Trends Neurosci* 1993;16:460–5.

Haan MN, Aiello AE, West NA, Jagust WJ. C-reactive protein and rate of dementia in carriers and non carriers of Apolipoprotein APOE4 genotype. *Neurobiol Aging* 2008; 29:1774–82.

Hardy J. Pathways to primary neurodegenerative disease. *Ann NY Acad Sci* 2000;924:29–34.

Harold D, Abraham R, Hollingworth P et al. Genome-wide association study identifies variants at CLU and PICALM associated with Alzheimer's disease. *Nat Genet* 2009;Sep 6 [Epub ahead of print]

Hye A, Lynham S, Thambisetty M et al. Proteome-based plasma biomarkers for Alzheimer's disease. *Brain* 2006;129:3042–50.

Licastro F, Chiappelli M. Brain immune responses cognitive decline and dementia: relationship with phenotype expression and genetic background. *Mech Ageing Dev* 2003;124:539–48.

Mattson MP, Chan SL, Duan W. Modification of brain aging and neurodegenerative disorders by genes, diet, and behavior. *Physiol Rev* 2002;82:637–72.

Mattson MP. Infectious agents and age-related neurodegenerative disorders. *Ageing Res Rev* 2004; 3:105–20.

Mattson MP. Modification of ion homeostasis by lipid peroxidation: roles in neuronal degeneration and adaptive plasticity. *Trends Neurosci* 1998;21:53–7.

Mattson MP. Oxidative stress, perturbed calcium homeostasis, and immune dysfunction in Alzheimer's disease. *J Neurovirol* 2002;8:539–50.

Moreira PI, Zhu X, Lee HG et al. The (un)balance between metabolic and oxidative abnormalities and cellular compensatory responses in Alzheimer disease. *Mech Ageing Dev* 2006;127:501–6.

O'Brien JT, Erkinjuntti T, Reisberg B et al. Vascular cognitive impairment. *Lancet Neurol* 2003;2:89–98.

Parachikova A, Agadjanyan MG, Cribbs DH et al. Inflammatory changes parallel the early stages of Alzheimer disease. *Neurobiol Aging* 2007;28:1821–33.

Purandare N, Burns A, Daly KJ et al. Cerebral emboli as a potential cause of Alzheimer's disease and vascular dementia: case-control study. *BMJ* 2006;332:1119–24.

Rea TD, Breitner JC, Psaty BM et al. Statin use and the risk of incident dementia: the Cardiovascular Health Study. *Arch Neurol* 2005;62:1047–51.

Reitz C, Bos MJ, Hofman A et al. Prestroke cognitive performance, incident stroke, and risk of dementia: the Rotterdam Study. *Stroke* 2008;39:36–41.

Ritchie CW, Bush AI, Mackinnon A et al. Metal-protein attenuation with iodochlorhydroxyquin (clioquinol) targeting Abeta amyloid deposition and toxicity in Alzheimer disease: a pilot phase 2 clinical trial. *Arch Neurol* 2003;60:1685–91.

Roses AD. Causes or consequences of inflammation and pathological signs of Alzheimer disease. *Neurobiol Aging* 2000;21:423–5.

Selkoe DJ. Alzheimer's disease: genes, proteins, and therapy. *Physiol Rev* 2001; 81:741–66.

Sparks DL, Sabbagh MN, Breitner JC et al. Is cholesterol a culprit in Alzheimer's disease? *Int Psychogeriatr* 2003;15 (suppl 1):153–9.

Szekely CA, Breitner JC, Fitzpatrick AL et al. NSAID use and dementia risk in the Cardiovascular Health Study: role of APOE and NSAID type. *Neurology* 2008;70: 17–24.

Troncoso JC, Zonderman AB, Resnick SM et al. Effect of infarcts on dementia in the Baltimore longitudinal study of aging. *Ann Neurol* 2008;64:168–76.

Tschanz JT, Corcoran C, Skoog I et al. Dementia: the leading predictor of death in a defined elderly population: the Cache County Study. *Neurology* 2004;62:1156–62.

Tunstall N, Owen MJ, Williams J et al. Familial influence on variation in age of onset and behavioural phenotype in Alzheimer's disease. *Br J Psychiatry* 2000; 176:156–9.

10 Future treatments

In Chapter 7 we described prescription treatments that may improve the cognitive performance of people with dementia. As we noted, there are currently good arguments for the cost–benefit advantage of these drugs, but the advantage would be greater still if we could develop a means to identify the individual patients who would respond. A corollary problem is the measurement of response in individual patients, and evaluation of their 'responder' versus 'non-responder' status. While some patients show a distinct improvement with an acetylcholinesterase (AChE) inhibitor or memantine, most show either a subtle improvement in their sense of mental focus and facility, or no change at all. Even the last of these is difficult to evaluate because of the inherently progressive nature of Alzheimer's dementia, so that the clinician may be left to wonder how the patient would have fared without treatment. Thus, the common dilemma: when to stop, or at least change to a different agent. A solution to this difficulty could save huge amounts of money that are essentially wasted on giving AChE inhibitors to (perhaps) 50% of patients whose well-being is not being improved by these agents.

We need to improve methods for dealing with this issue, which can present in at least two forms. Clinicians may take on patients with dementia who are already receiving AChE inhibitor treatment, and whose family reports that the drug 'is helping', but cannot elaborate. Alternatively, a clinician initiates treatment with an AChE inhibitor but is unsure of any benefit. In neither situation do we have a widely accepted protocol for testing the effect of treatment cessation. To aggravate matters, some experienced doctors have witnessed at least one instance of a patient experiencing a precipitous, even irreversible, decline in function when treatment with an AChE inhibitor is stopped. We therefore need to develop ways to terminate treatments with expectation of doing no harm, so long as the treatments are re-initiated when needed. Clearly, such a protocol will require close medical or nursing supervision, probably including the frequent (weekly?) administration of structured observation scales to assess cognitive and functional abilities.

A number of treatments currently in development are targeted at the so-called amyloid cascade hypothesis of Alzheimer's disease. Most of these have encountered safety difficulties or have shown disappointing results otherwise.

At the time of writing, there is considerable interest in a novel treatment approach using an 'old-fashioned' anti-histamine drug called dimebon, which, in one well-designed and well-executed clinical trial, was shown to produce substantial improvement in the function of patients with Alzheimer's disease. Further evaluation of the safety and efficacy of this drug is required.

Rather less has been done to date with drugs that target the phosphorylation of tau protein or the dissolution of ordinarily insoluble tau aggregates. This pathway is will be become of greater interest as we learn more about the relevance of tangle pathology as an important correlate of neurodegeneration in Alzheimer's disease.

We also need a way to explain why non-steroidal anti-inflammatory drugs (NSAIDs) have frequently appeared to be associated with a reduced incidence of Alzheimer's dementia, but in several trials have been shown to have a modest effect or no effect as a treatment for established disease. Compounding this problem are the recently discovered cardiovascular risks of NSAIDs (most notably selective COX-2 inhibitors, but all prescription NSAIDs in the USA now carry a 'black box' safety warning about these risks). The only randomized trial to assess the efficacy of NSAIDs for the prevention of Alzheimer's dementia was stopped early because of this type of safety issue. Published results from the few years during which participants were receiving treatments did not show benefit, but this is perhaps not surprising since considerable epidemiological data show no real effect of these drugs when taken in the last few years before dementia onset. Follow-up results from this trial will be of considerable interest.

The example of NSAIDs underscores one final point: ultimately, it is the prevention of dementia and Alzheimer's disease that is wanted, not necessarily its treatment. Not only does dementia usually reflect advanced brain damage; it may also be true that by this time the disease process has advanced to a point of resistance to any intervention, rendering it difficult even to arrest the progression of symptoms. Whereas efforts over the past two decades have concentrated on treatment or disease modification, in more recent years interest has evolved towards greater interest in the identification of prodromal Alzheimer's disease and possible interventions to prevent the 'conversion' of this condition to dementia – although results to date have been largely disappointing. So far, there has been some skepticism about the potential for developing primary prevention strategies through prevention trials, because of their high cost and lengthy duration. A more recent development that may circumvent some of these difficulties is the identification of 'biomarkers' that can indicate the neurodegenerative process of Alzheimer's disease. An example of such an approach is the measurement of soluble Aβ and tau in cerebrospinal fluid, or the ratio of these measures. While it is unlikely that these sorts of measures can satisfy the demanding criteria for a 'surrogate marker' for disease (such as CD4 count or viral load in HIV/AIDS), they can at least offer encouragement during the long march of prevention trials, perhaps even preventing their abandonment for 'futility'. There are enormous potential problems in the conduct of prevention trials, which Donald Fredrickson, former director of the US National Institutes of Health, referred to as "the indispensible ordeal". To quote Fredrickson further, however, considering the potential benefits against the difficulties in the conduct of such trials, "have we really any choice?"

Useful addresses

UK

Alzheimer Scotland
Helpline: 0808 808 3000
Tel: +44 (0)131 243 1453
www.alzscot.org

Alzheimer's Research Trust
Tel: +44 (0)1223 843899
www.alzheimers-research.org.uk

Alzheimer's Society
Helpline: 0845 300 0336
Tel: +44 (0)20 7423 3500
www.alzheimers.org.uk

Carers UK
Tel: +44 (0)20 7490 8818
www.carersuk.org

Dementia Research Centre
Tel: +44 (0)20 7829 8773
http://dementia.ion.ucl.ac.uk

The Royal College of Psychiatrists
Tel: +44 (0)20 7235 2351
www.rcpsych.ac.uk

USA

Alzheimer's Association
Helpline: 1 800 272 3900
Tel: +1 312 335 8700
www.alz.org

Alzheimer's Disease Education and Referral (ADEAR) Center
Toll-free: 1 800 438 4380
www.nia.nih.gov/alzheimers

American Psychiatric Association
Tel: +1 703 907 7300
www.psych.org

International

Alzheimer Europe
Tel: 352 297 970
www.alzheimer-europe.org

Alzheimer Research Forum
www.alzforum.org

Alzheimer's Australia
Helpline: 1 800 100 500
Tel: +61 (0)2 6254 4233
www.alzheimers.org.au

Alzheimer's Disease International
Tel: +44 (0)20 7981 0880
www.alz.co.uk

Alzheimer Society of Canada
Toll-free: 1 800 616 8816
Tel: +1 416 488 8772
www.alzheimer.ca

World Psychiatric Association
www.wpanet.org

Index